The Far-Reaching Benefits of Infant Massage

Infant massage, as it is shared in this book, is not a fad. It is an ancient art that connects you deeply with the person who is your baby, and it helps you to understand your baby's particular nonverbal language and respond with love and respectful listening. It empowers you as a parent, for it gives you the means by which you become an expert on your own child and therefore can respond according to your baby's unique needs. Rather than growing up selfish and demanding (though all kids go through such stages), a child whose voice is heard, whose heart is full, and who is enveloped in love overflows with that love and naturally, unselfconsciously gives of himself to others. He learns what healthy, respectful touch is by being touched that way. He learns self-discipline by watching his parents and imitating them. The deep emotional bonds formed in infancy lay a foundation for a lifetime of trust, courage, dependability, faith, and love.

"Vimala McClure is a visionary who has helped innumerable people become far better parents. She has become my own personal Dr. Spock, the main source I turn to for loving and competent guidance and inspiration in raising my children."

— MARC ALLEN, author of *Visionary Business* and *A Visionary Life*

"What a brilliant way to love and nurture a child! The first connection between parent and child is physical, through the body. By using the techniques that Vimala has developed, your parental relationship will be off to a magnificent start."

— JUDY FORD, author of *Wonderful Ways to Love a Child* and *Wonderful Ways to Be a Family*

"Embodying spirit is the work of our times . . . and the beautiful, empowering words of Vimala McClure bring to our everyday life a deep and abiding experience of the timeliness of the body, soul, and spirit. We are changed."

— CAROLYN CRAFT, director of Wisdom Radio

By Vimala McClure

Infant Massage: A Handbook for Loving Parents

A Woman's Guide to Tantra Yoga

The Tao of Motherhood

Bangladesh: Rivers in a Crowded Land

The Path of Parenting: Twelve Principles to Guide Your Journey

Teaching Infant Massage: A Handbook for Instructors

Infant Massage

Infant Massage

A Handbook for Loving Parents

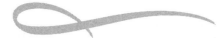

Vimala McClure

Fourth Edition

Bantam Books   New York

2017 Bantam Books Trade Paperback Edition

Copyright © 1979, 1982, 1989, 2000, 2017 by Vimala McClure

Photographs copyright © 2000 by Vimala McClure

Published in the United States by Bantam Books, an imprint of Random House,
a division of Penguin Random House LLC, New York.

BANTAM BOOKS and the HOUSE colophon are registered
trademarks of Penguin Random House LLC.

Originally published by Monterey Laboratories, Inc. in 1979. Revised editions were
published in trade paperback by Bantam Books, an imprint of Random House,
a division of Penguin Random House LLC, in 1982, 1989, and 2000.

Portions of Chapters 10 and 12 appeared in *Mothering* magazine
(September 1986 and Spring 1987).

Photograph on page 251 appeared in the 1982 edition.

LIBRARY OF CONGRESS CATALOGING-IN-PUBLICATION DATA
Names: McClure, Vimala Schneider.
Title: Infant massage : a handbook for loving parents / Vimala Schneider McClure.
Description: Fourth revised edition. | New York : Bantam, [2017]
Identifiers: LCCN 2016043579| ISBN 9781101965948 (paperback) |
ISBN 9780425286678 (ebook)
Subjects: LCSH: Massage for infants—Handbooks, manuals, etc. | BISAC:
FAMILY & RELATIONSHIPS / Life Stages / Infants & Toddlers. | FAMILY &
RELATIONSHIPS / Parenting / General. | HEALTH & FITNESS /
Massage & Reflexotherapy.
Classification: LCC RJ61 .M48 2017 | DDC 618.92/02—dc23 LC record available at
lccn.loc.gov/2016043579

Printed in the United States of America on acid-free paper

randomhousebooks.com

2 4 6 8 9 7 5 3 1

Book design by Donna Sinisgalli

Dedicated to P. R. Sarkar and to my beloved children

Contents

Acknowledgments   xi

Foreword: A Gift of Touch, by Peggy O'Mara   xv

Preface by Stephen Berman, M.D., F.A.A.P.   xix

Introduction   xxi

Chapter 1: Why Massage Your Baby?   3

Chapter 2: Your Baby's Sensory World   11

Chapter 3: The Importance of Skin Stimulation   21

Chapter 4: Stress and Relaxation   31

Chapter 5: Bonding, Attachment, and Infant Massage   37

Chapter 6: The Elements of Bonding   45

Chapter 7: Attachment and the Benefits of Infant Massage   65

Chapter 8: Especially for Fathers   79

Chapter 9: Helping Baby (and You) Learn to Relax   87

Chapter 10: Your Baby's Brain   95

Chapter 11: Music and Massage   105

Chapter 12: Getting Ready   113

Chapter 13: How to Massage Your Baby   125

Chapter 14: Crying, Fussing, and Other Baby Language   181
(Including Cues, Reflexes, and Behavioral States)

Chapter 15: Minor Illness and Colic   203

Chapter 16: Your Premature Baby   215

Chapter 17: Your Baby with Special Needs   227

Chapter 18: Your Growing Child and Sibling Bonding   237
Through Massage

Chapter 19: Your Adopted or Foster Children   255

Chapter 20: A Note to Teen Parents   265

Resources   271

References and Recommendations   277

Acknowledgments

Heartfelt thanks to all those who have helped and supported my work over the years. Special thanks to the following people for helping bring this new edition to birth: to Elana Seplow-Jolley and Richard Callison for making it happen; to all the instructors and trainers in the International Association of Infant Massage (IAIM) for their input, experience, and support; and to Peggy O'Mara, former editor and publisher of *Mothering* magazine, who started her work just about the time I did and has been a great inspiration to me all these years.

I thank my friends and colleagues in the International Association of Infant Massage for their hard work, dedication, and service to humanity through this work. It is their realization of its long-range potential that has brought its benefits to so many parents worldwide and, I believe, contributed to a significant change in our infant parenting practices and the way we respond to infants' needs.

Thanks to trainer Clara Ute Zacher Laves and her husband, Markus Zacher, for helping with the photographs, and to infant massage instructor Joni Rubinstein and her teen parents for helping get those photographs done and being so conscientious in doing so.

I also want to acknowledge my sister Madhi Shirman, whose encouragement supported me to begin teaching infant massage in the first place, and whose unwavering support of my work has meant the world to me.

The photographer who took the beautiful photos in Chapter 13 as well as some others is Gunter Kiepke. Thank you, Gunter; you did the most wonderful job and far exceeded my expectations!

In the process of putting this book together, I gathered many, many photos and was unable to use more than a quarter of the total I had to choose from. I want to thank all the parents and babies who allowed me to photograph them or have other photographers do it for me. I may accidentally leave out a name in the following list, if the photos were taken elsewhere and I can't find the name, or so long ago I can't remember which release goes with which name. But please know I am very grateful to everyone who contributed in any way; by doing so, you have contributed to the well-being of future generations.

The people who graciously allowed me to use their photographs (which may or may not appear in this book):

Maraliz Bracamonte, Naidelyn Alvarez
Andrea Bassett, Deondre Beckwith
Bridgett Washington, Allezae Brown
Gabriel De La Luz, Christina Hogbin, Gabriel De La Luz Jr.
Shenika Evans, Shavel Evans
Yvette Hernandez, Juliette Contreras
Alexandria Boney
Anke D. Bahr, Lenja Kim
Oliver Fuchs
Corinna Reissner, Anna Catharina
Susan Whittlesey, Anne Young
Nancy Duffy, Nicole Green
Susan Pressel, Justin Pressel
Marlene Stieha, Analeesa Stieha
Gina Kincaid, Elaina Marie Santa Cruz
Cindy Shelton, Christina Shelton
Jan Lapetino and baby
Heidi Dorsey, Tia Dorsey, Carlos Dorsey
Mary Foster, Lance Foster, Michael Foster
Clara Ute Zacher Laves
Gabriela Silva, Jasline Ariana Garcia

Thanks to the wonderful certified instructors and trainers for IAIM around the world who graciously sent me photographs for this new edition:

Jody Wright

Andreina Di Geronimo Bustamante

Mercedes DelCastillo

Juliana Dellinger-Bavolek

Ana Lucia Penagos

Valentina Scarfone

Foreword

A Gift of Touch

In the summer of 1974, when my first child was born, I didn't know anything about infant massage, but I knew that I wanted to touch my baby. It was a hot summer, and it felt good to carry my daughter around skin to skin. I would take her outside and lay her on a blanket in the fresh air under the eaves of our house. There I would rub her with sweet almond oil and massage her soft skin.

At about this same time, a few hundred miles away, Vimala was massaging her babies. Vimala is the premier proponent of infant massage in the world, and was among the first to write about massage in general and infant massage in particular. In fact, Vimala's work in infant massage has been instrumental in the birth of touch therapy and bodywork in the United States and has helped to popularize and legitimize massage throughout the world. Her early work on infant massage and premature babies was years ahead of its time and continues to influence the humane care of newborns through touch.

For many of us, infant massage has been a way to learn to touch our babies and to become comfortable with touch in general. Those of us who became parents in the 1960s and 1970s grew up in much less intimate and "touchy-feely" times than today. Seeing people hugging affectionately in public as we do today was almost unheard of forty years ago, when Vimala's innocent book sparked a revolution in touch in the United States.

As revolutionary as it is, infant massage is really an old-fashioned idea, and its beauty lies in the fact that anyone can do it. It's simple and it's good for you. It can't hurt you or your baby and it costs nothing. Don't think that you need special skills or talents to massage your baby. It comes naturally and is a way for our babies to teach us about themselves and for us to learn how to touch.

Touch is as necessary to the human baby as food. Anthropologist Margaret Mead studied tribal societies all over the world and found that the most violent tribes were those that withheld touch in infancy. Neurologist Richard Restak says that physically holding and carrying an infant turn out to be the most important factors responsible for the infant's normal mental and social development. The effects of this normal development do not just influence infancy but impact the neural and neuroendocrine functions underlying emotional behavior in enduring ways. In other words, the more we experience authentic intimacy as infants, the more we are capable of intimacy as adults. And what could be more intimate than gentle touch?

Research at the University of Miami Miller School of Medicine suggests that massage can stimulate nerves in the brain that facilitate food absorption, resulting in faster weight gain. Massage can lower stress hormones, resulting in improved immune function. Touch therapy can also help premature infants gain weight faster, asthmatic children improve breathing function, diabetic children comply with treatment, and sleepless babies fall asleep more easily. Other research indicates that touch therapy can benefit infants and children with eczema and can improve parent-baby interactions.

What better way to improve parent-baby interactions, what better way to ensure your baby is getting enough skin-to-skin contact, than with infant massage? The soothing oil and the soft, easy touch of your hands are sensory delights that you can share with your baby as you introduce him to the world. Massage is such a nice way to get to know your baby and to spend time together in the early weeks and months. Soon enough she will be up and around, and these touch times of the early months will be sweet memories.

There were eight years between those first massages I gave my daughter and the first real massage I had myself. It was not until the 1980s that massage therapists were easily available, and it took me many years to become comfortable with the idea of "indulging" in massage. Something that at first seemed frivolous to me has now become a cornerstone of my health care. Vimala has taught us that touch is not a self-indulgence but is actually a basic human need. How unfortunate that we would consider fulfilling such a basic need to be self-indulgent.

I would recommend that you spoil your children with the indulgence of your touch. Perhaps there is nothing quite so personal and intimate as the gift of infant massage. Like parenthood in general, infant massage enriches the parent as well as the baby. It establishes a tradition of touch that will enhance your relationship with your child for years to come.

Peggy O'Mara

Former editor and publisher, *Mothering*

Preface

During the past several decades, physicians have reassessed the importance of maternal-infant bonding in relation to development. Studies at the University of Colorado and elsewhere have demonstrated that infants whose mothers have difficulty in touching, cuddling, or talking to them during the first few months of life are more likely to suffer from developmental growth or delay. Scientific advances in the understanding of the newborn and infant sensory, motor, and cognitive processes have resulted in new appreciation for many of the cultural parenting practices of the nonindustrialized world. For example, infant carrier packs such as the Snugli are modeled after practices observed in many parts of Africa and Latin America. These infant carriers promote mutual feelings of comfort and security associated with close body contact and still provide the parent freedom of movement.

In *Infant Massage: A Handbook for Loving Parents,* Vimala McClure introduces us to a form of parenting that has been practiced for centuries in India. The value of infant massage as a parenting technique can be appreciated best by recognizing the maternal-infant interaction as displayed in the faces of parents and babies shown in the pictures in this book. Hopefully, parents will accept infant massage into the American way of life in the same way that Lamaze childbirth classes and infant carriers have been accepted. An added plus to infant massage is the opportunity it provides for the father, especially of a breastfed baby, to have positive interaction with his child.

I am a pediatrician, and the best advice I can give you is to try the techniques in this book. If the interaction between you and your child is enjoyable and the massage is fun, you will be providing your infant with a pleasurable form of stimulation that may build a strong foundation for your child's development.

Stephen Berman, M.D., F.A.A.P.

Former president, American Academy of Pediatrics

Director, Center for Global Health, University of
   Colorado School of Public Health

Section Head in General Academic Pediatrics,
   Children's Hospital Colorado

Introduction

In 1973, I was twenty-one years old. I had been practicing yoga and meditation for a few years, and I wanted to be a yoga instructor. The only way to do that, at the time, was to travel to a training center in northwest India. The training center was also an orphanage; I was expected to work in the orphanage by day, and train with a yoga monk by night. There were three Indian girls in their teens who were going to become yoga nuns.

During the time I was there, I made a discovery that would substantially redirect my life. I loved the children, who always came rushing to me, wanting to hug me, to sit on my lap, and for me to sing with them. I noticed that all the children I saw, both in and out of the orphanage, were delightful. They were open and relaxed and always smiling. In spite of their extreme poverty, they were happy, they had a relaxed way of being in the world, and I often saw boys—not just girls—walking around with a baby on their hips.

One night after class, I was walking around the compound, looking up at the stars, which were so bright and different from what I saw in America. I approached the sleeping quarters of the children and peeked in. A girl, about twelve years old, was massaging a baby and singing softly. I waited until she was finished, and went in to talk to her. Luckily, I knew some Bengali—her language. She told me that massage, especially for babies, was traditional. An Indian mother regularly massages everyone in her family and passes these techniques on to her daughters. At the orphanage, the eldest massage the little ones nearly every day. I asked her if she could show me how to do it. She happily agreed, and allowed me to massage the baby, who was so relaxed and sleepy. I learned how to use oil, warm my hands, and perform each stroke. The baby connected with me immediately. She gazed into my eyes, smiled, and drifted off to sleep.

I was profoundly touched by this experience. I thought about it a lot. I began to think that maybe the children in India were so relaxed in the way they carried themselves because they had been massaged every day in their infancy. It was a type of nurturing I hadn't seen in the United States. I received its benefits when, during my last week in India, I succumbed to malaria. When I was delirious with fever, all the women in the neighborhood came to look after me. They massaged my body with practiced hands, as if I were a baby, and they sang to me, taking turns until my fever broke. I will never forget the feeling of their hands and hearts touching me.

On my way to the train station after a tearful good-bye at the orphanage, my rickshaw stopped to let a buffalo cart go by. To my right was a shanty—just a few boards and some canvas—where a family lived by the road. A young mother sat in the dirt with her baby across her knees, lovingly massaging him and singing. As I watched her, I thought, "There is so much more to life than material wealth." She had so little, yet she could offer her baby this beautiful gift of love and security, a gift that would help to make him a compassionate human being.

I thought about all the children I had known in India, and how loving, warm, and playful they were in spite of their so-called disadvantages. They took care of one another, and they accepted responsibility without reservation. Perhaps, I thought, they are able to be so loving, so relaxed and natural because they have been loved like this as infants, and infants have been loved this way in India for thousands of years. Massage, perhaps, makes them at home in their world, not enemies or conquerors of it. It welcomes them to the warmth and love that are here for them, allowing them to retain the gentle spirit that comes clothed in a new, still unformed, and fragile body. And it helps that body adjust to the stimulation of a world full of noises, lights, movement, sharpness, and clamor with curiosity, not fear. Later I learned from many mothers and grandmothers this ancient art of heart and hands that so clearly impacts the bodies, minds, and spirits of the people who receive it.

Though I had noticed how cuddly, relaxed, and friendly the Indian children seemed, it wasn't until I became pregnant a few years later that I started seriously thinking about the benefits of infant massage. During my pregnancy, I developed an interest in all aspects of childbirth and infant development, and began studying everything I could find. I read the book *Touching* by Ashley Montagu, and I grew determined to integrate massage into my baby's life every day.

As I thought about how to do this and read about the incredible importance of nurturing touch to all mammals, I studied Montagu's bibliography and decided to find the research upon which his claims were based. I had a feeling that this information could be translated to humans. Montagu had made the connection throughout his book, and thinking about massaging my baby was suddenly very exciting.

I spent most of my pregnancy driving from our home in Boulder, Colorado, to the big medical library in neighboring Denver. I made copies of every single piece of research in Montagu's book and brought them home. The more I learned about how animal mothers supply nurturing touch to their infants, and its crucial importance, the more excited I became. For example, cats have rough tongues and lick their newborns like crazy. Everybody thinks it is to get them clean. But actually, they are massaging the babies to help their internal processes work, such as respiration, digestion, and circulation. Without that, the kittens die. I had read about failure to thrive, when human babies get depressed and spiral downward even though they are receiving the best nutrition; when they lack nurturing touch, they begin to die. That was an "aha" moment for me.

My first child was born in September 1976, and I began massaging him every day. Having taught yoga for several years, I found that a number of its massage techniques and poses were easily incorporated into our daily massage routine—a routine based on my own combination of ancient Indian and modern Swedish methods along with techniques I knew as a yoga instructor. This joyful blend provided my son with a wonderful balance of outgoing and incoming energy, of tension release and stimulation. Additionally, it seemed to relieve the painful gas he experienced that first month. Gentle yoga-like exercises ended our massage playfully and further helped in toning and relieving his digestive system.

I began massaging my baby immediately after he was born. You would think that all was roses and rainbows, but that was not the case. He had colic and was miserable, crying for hours at a time. He accepted the massage, but when I started massaging his belly, he would fuss and sometimes cry.

Most parents would probably stop, assuming that he just "didn't like" being massaged. I had the hunch, in part due to my research, that his colic was simply a result of an underdeveloped gastrointestinal system. I comforted him, but didn't stop massaging. I thought about how the digestive system works, and I thought about yoga postures that I knew were created especially for irritable bowel syndrome, to help relieve gas trapped in the colon.

I began changing the strokes I had learned in India. I had several massage therapist friends, and asked them to show me what they would do with a client experiencing these problems. I even got several massages myself, so that I could experience what the movements felt like. I designed a series of strokes that combined traditional Indian massage, whose strokes move from the center of the body outward to aid in releasing tension, with Swedish massage techniques, whose strokes move toward the heart to aid in circulation. I added some reflexology and modified yoga postures. Within two weeks, my son's colic had disappeared.

By the time my baby was about five months old, I had developed a routine that I turned into a curriculum for a five-session course. I wanted to share this wonderful art with other parents. I made a little flyer and asked local businesses to display it on their counters and in their windows. My first class was with five mothers and their babies in the front room of our little apartment. Since then, thousands of parents and infants have attended my classes and sought private instruction. Over the years, they have provided me with continual education and inspiration, for which I am most grateful.

In May 1977, Frédérick Leboyer's book *Loving Hands,* a poetic observation of a woman in India massaging her baby, was published. The world was ready for infant massage, a term I coined myself. There was a huge surge of interest in pregnancy, birth, and babies. Drs. John Kennell and Marshall Klaus did research on bonding, which became the topic of the day. Once I began looking into bonding, I discovered that all of the elements known to help with bonding were part of infant massage. So massage was a way to continue the bonding process with both parents in the fourth trimester and beyond.

Soon I had fifteen to eighteen mothers and babies coming to classes (fathers would come later) that I taught twice a week. I began to make handouts for them, instructing them how to prepare for the massage, recommending books, and showing research, and I came up with a feedback form for them to fill out in the last class. Every possible type of mother and baby attended my classes; I learned so much in those early years.

In the years since my first classes, interest in infant massage has exploded around the world among parents and professionals alike. In 1978, I wrote a manuscript that I called *Infant Massage: A Handbook for Loving Parents.* Through many magical moments, it was published by Bantam Books of New York.

I began training instructors, then trained trainers to train instructors. We now have an international nonprofit organization, the first and largest of its kind, for the preservation and dissemination of this ancient practice: the International Association of Infant Massage, with instructors in more than seventy countries. Many hospitals now train nursery staff to use massage and holding techniques with premature and sick babies and offer instruction to parents in an effort to promote bonding and ease babies' discomforts. In addition, the benefits of this simple tradition, intuitively developed and refined in the

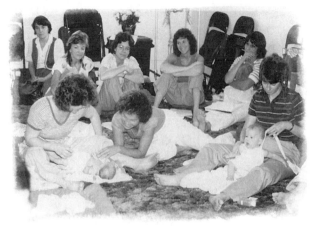

"laboratories" of thousands of years of human experience, are being recognized day by day in modern scientific research. (I have met with many a joke in this regard, teased gently as a Westerner who needs double-blind studies to prove that grass grows if you water it!)

My children are grown now, and the impact of our experience with massage during their infancies has not diminished. The daily massages provided a foundation for physical, emotional, and spiritual harmony and closeness that we all carry with us for life.

I would like to share a letter I received from a mother who learned infant massage from this book when I first began teaching. It is not meant as medical advice; certainly if your baby has medical problems, you should work with your medical professionals and be sure the massage you deliver is appropriate for your baby's needs. I share it with you to show you how profoundly this simple practice can affect a family. I thank the mother who sent me this priceless letter.

Dear Vimala,

I wanted to personally write and thank you for the invaluable contribution you made to my children.

My son was born addicted to a drug that I had been given to stop seizures from toxemia and premature labor. Additionally, I was treated several times with other intravenous drugs. Throughout the pregnancy, repeated physicians scolded me and my husband for continuing the pregnancy. We were assured that our baby would be handicapped, a "vegetable," and so on. We fought hard and well as he survived to thirty-eight weeks gestation, born at a robust eight pounds, fifteen ounces. It was soon obvious that his nervous system was badly affected by the drugs and stress.

He cried endlessly or slept nonstop, missing feedings. If he was startled, his little arms and legs would jut out and shake uncontrollably. The doctors suggested more drugs to calm him. They again asserted that his nervous system and probably his brain were irreparably harmed. A wonderful neighbor and breastfeeding professional came to our rescue.

She taught me your methods of infant massage to calm him and showed me how to swaddle him to prevent jarring his sensitive nervous system. To make a long story a tad bit shorter, he grew to be an inquisitive and absolutely delightful toddler. The shaking subsided, and a brilliant intellect came forth combined with an energy that was tiring to us poor adults. Today, my supposedly "handicapped" child is in college, a National Merit Scholar, a recognized leader, a wonderful volunteer worker, and engaged to be married to a dynamic and equally bright young woman. He was nationally recognized as a teen and was offered more than $375,000 in scholarships. He works with severely handicapped adults and plans on being a physician.

My second son was also the product of a terribly high-risk pregnancy. Drug therapies were a bit more advanced and, with the help of diet, controlled the toxemia. He was born with noted neurological deficits. By the age of five months, we were cautioned that he had begun to show the symptoms of autism. He was highly irritable and, to put it simply, a challenging baby.

I once again drew on my experience with massage. The tension in his little limbs would melt away, and he remained in contact with the world. I kept him close to me, leaving him only with caregivers for short periods of time who were willing to comfort him as needed, to hold him, massage him. Though still plagued with a few problems, he is a very bright and caring sixteen-year-old. He is already doing computer design for toy and software companies.

Without the help of my neighbor who had studied your techniques, I do not believe that either of these young men would be where they are today. I believe that their intellectual, physical, and emotional development is attributable to the comfort they received as infants. How can I ever thank you? Please know that this mother will be in your debt forever.

Sincerely,
A grateful mother

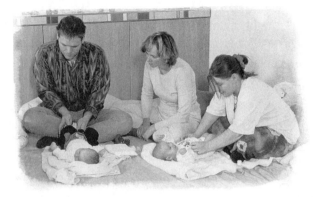

Infant massage can promote the kind of parenting that this attentive mother was able to provide. Its benefits go far beyond the immediate physiological gains. As you massage your baby regularly, you will discover that you develop a bond with your child that will last a lifetime.

On Choosing the Right Word

Like many authors, I have encountered the male-female pronoun problem. When referring to a baby, do I say "he or she"? Or "he/she"? Or "s/he"? All of these seem clumsy and forced. So to get my own message across as simply as possible, I have chosen to refer to the baby as "he" some of the time and "she" some of the time—providing balance for all.

Another problem is in reference to the person massaging the baby. I have used "mother" much of the time as the primary masseuse in the book, both for the sake of convenience and because, in my experience, she is most often principally involved in this care. In addition, massage, as I see it, is a "mothering" activity, whether it is performed by mother or father, brother or sister, grandma or grandpa.

Since it is my sincere hope that fathers may be equally interested and involved, I have included a special section for them. To those fathers who read the book in its entirety and decide to massage their babies, I would simply ask them to change "mother" to "father" in their minds at the appropriate places.

About References

Throughout the book, I cite research about various topics. I have decided not to footnote the book so that it doesn't read like a thesis. I've tried to note the research in the "References and Recommendations" section, but I've probably missed a few of the studies I refer to in the book.

Enough said!

Infant Massage

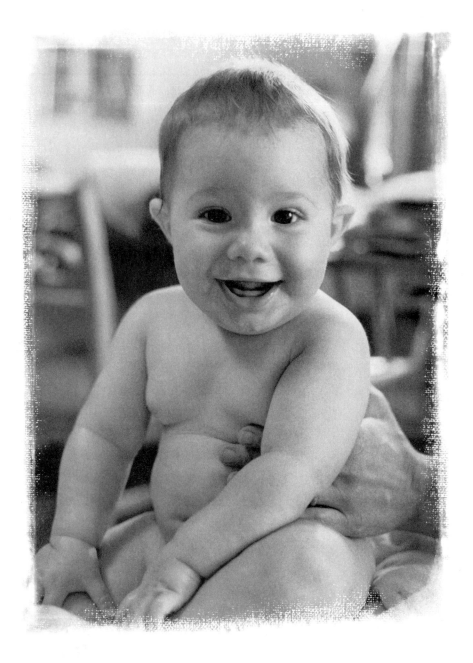

Chapter 1

Why Massage Your Baby?

Being touched and caressed,
being massaged,
is food for the infant.
Food as necessary
as minerals, vitamins, and proteins.

—DR. FRÉDÉRICK LEBOYER

An Age-Old Tradition

A young mother gently cradles her baby in her lap as the afternoon sun streams through cracks in the wooden door. For the second time that day, she carefully removes the tiny cap and begins to unwrap the swaddling bands of soft white linen and wool.

Freed from his snug encasement, the baby kicks and waves his little arms, listening to the now-familiar *swish-swish* of the warm oil in his mother's hands and the comforting sound of her balmy lullaby. So begins his twice-daily massage. The scene is in a Jewish shtetl, one of the small enclaves in Poland in the early nineteenth century, but we could be anywhere in the world, in any century, for it is a familiar tableau of motherhood in every culture throughout the ages.

From the Eskimos of the Canadian Arctic to the Ganda of East Africa, from South India to Northern Ireland, in Russia, China, Sweden, and South America, in South Sea Islands huts and modern American homes, babies are lovingly massaged, caressed, and crooned to every day. Mothers all over the world know their babies need to be held, carried, rocked, and touched. The gentle art of infant massage has been part of baby caregiving traditions passed from parent to child for generations. Asked why, each culture would provide different answers. Most would simply say, "It is our custom."

Many of the family customs of our ancestors, turned aside in the early twentieth century in the interest of "progress," are returning to our lives as modern science rediscovers their importance and their contribution to our infants' well-being and that of whole communities. Cross-cultural studies have demonstrated that in societies where infants are held, massaged, rocked, breastfed, and carried, adults are less aggressive and violent, more cooperative and compassionate. Our great-great-grandmothers would stand up and utter a great "I told you so!" were they to observe our "new" discoveries in infant care.

Before your baby is born, you may envision yourself calmly and blissfully being a parent, or you may be terrified that you don't know what to do with this new human depending on you for its very existence. It is fairly easy now, with the Internet, to read a lot about infants—what they need, what they don't need, how to provide the best environment for them, how to respond to their cries and fusses, and so on.

Scientific research has blossomed over the past decades, and many of the parenting styles of our grandparents' day have been proven to be almost barbaric. Figure out how to both take care of yourself and provide your infant with the love, attention, and healthy environment that she desperately needs. Those who say, "Well, I turned out all right! The way my parents did it will work for me," don't recognize the many problems and the physical, mental, and emotional health risks they faced or will face because of how they were raised.

If you can be firmly rooted in who you are, you will find that you can intuit the right decisions as you live with your baby. You will make mistakes, but as you relax, slow down, empower yourself with good information, and have confidence in who you are, you can correct your course as you go along. In this way, no permanent damage is done. Your child responds to you "being yourself." Trying to parent in some way that isn't coming from your deepest principles is confusing for your child, and damaging in the long term.

Only you can decide, according to what feels best to you, whether you give birth at home or in a hospital or birthing center; choose to immunize or not, breastfeed or not; whether your children wear exclusively natural fibers or not; whether or not you choose day care; how you discipline and communicate with a toddler; and so on. After doing your own research about the issues, make your decisions from a deep inner place that makes you feel like a good parent, instead of simply going with what your parents tell you or with the current cultural flow.

Over and over again, it has been shown that the current cultural flow is often wrong. At one time it was common and accepted to give babies opium to keep them quiet. At one time mothers were told to wear masks and not to breathe on their babies or breastfeed them for fear of "contaminating" them. At one time parents were told not to respond to infants' cries for fear of "spoiling" them. At one time it was widely believed that babies didn't feel pain and that they could not see or hear in the womb or for the first weeks of life. Take the experts with a grain of salt, and listen to your own heart about what is right for you and your family.

Both for babies and parents, the benefits of infant massage are more far-reaching than may at first be obvious. For infants, massage is much more than a luxurious sensual experience. It is a tool for maintaining the child's health and well-being on many levels.

For parents, it is vital to feeling secure in your own ability to do something positive for—and get a positive response from—this squealing bit of newborn humanity suddenly and urgently put in your charge. It is not a therapy that you do *to* your baby; it is a deep communicative art that you do *with* your baby.

Can Babies Be Spoiled with Love and Attention?

Research can help us understand why traditional practices are so important. Knowing why, we are less quick to cast adrift customs that can deeply enrich our lives. Our concern about raising "spoiled" children comes from an earlier time when behaviorists, after discovering behavioral conditioning, thought that we could condition our babies to behave like little adults by ignoring their cries and not offering too much affection.

That approach eventually became popular again. (Fads swing like a pendulum from one extreme to another, and parenting advice is not immune to this phenomenon.) Popular baby care programs used to advise parents to put babies on rigid schedules, allow them to "cry it out" alone, and punish them for behavior that was not convenient for parents. The leaders of these movements also managed to convince parents that they damaged their infant's metabolism by breastfeeding on demand (despite all research to the contrary) and created spoiled, selfish children if parents responded to their needs and comforted them when they cried. Parents were admonished never to allow their infants to sleep with them, for they could easily kill them (again, despite all research to the contrary). These ideas represent a swing away from the natural parenting practices that had gained momentum in the 1970s and achieved recognition from pediatricians as healthy and normal by the 1990s. Here is a more practical and research-verified approach:

- In order to become well-adjusted, kind, empathic adults, babies require a lot of attention, affection, and response to their needs.
- Breastfeeding on demand, breast milk in a bottle, and bottle-feeding that emulates breastfeeding as closely as possible are essential to a baby's physical, mental, and emotional health as well as to continual bonding with parents.
- Cosleeping can easily be made completely safe if parents learn appropriate ways to make it happen.

Proof abounds that babies who are neglected and punished suffer bonding breaks and, without intervention, often grow up to be troubled if not antisocial or sociopathic, individuals. Since the mid-1970s, working with parents to bond more deeply with their infants, respect them, learn their nonverbal "language," and respond to them with love, I have received countless letters from parents saying infant massage changed their entire life as a family, and their children turned out to be lively, creative, inquisitive, secure, intelligent, social, loving, humanitarian human beings. I had this experience with my own two kids, now amazing adults; my own "laboratory" proved to me that my research and ideas are correct. Authoritarian advisers neglect to mention that parents all over the world have naturally responded with love to their babies, breastfed on demand, slept in "family beds," and carried infants in various types of slings for millennia—and that if you read the biographies of terrorists, serial killers, and cruel dictators, you will invariably find neglect or authoritarian treatment in childhood.

Infant massage, as it is shared in this book, is not a fad. It is an ancient art that connects you deeply with the person who is your baby, and it helps you to understand your baby's particular nonverbal language and respond with love and respectful listening. It empowers you as a parent, for it gives you the means by which you become an expert on your own child and therefore can respond according to your baby's unique needs. Rather than growing up selfish and demanding (though all kids go through such stages), a child whose voice is heard, whose heart is full, and who is enveloped in love overflows with that love and naturally, unselfconsciously gives of himself to others. He learns what healthy, respectful touch is by being touched that way. She learns self-discipline by watching her parents and imitating them. He has little to rebel against because there is no festering resentment of parents' authoritarian or autocratic, unpredictable rules and punishments. The deep emotional bonds formed in infancy lay a foundation for a lifetime of trust, courage, dependability, faith, and love.

Infant massage is not just for parents who embrace a certain lifestyle.

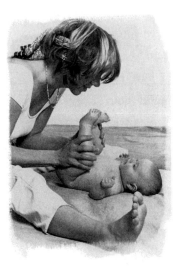

Whether your baby sleeps with you or in her own room, is breast- or bottle-fed, is weaned early or late—all these decisions are up to you. Massaging your baby simply communicates love, releases tension, and helps you better understand your baby's needs. The fact that it is fun is a wonderful added benefit!

After more than fifty years of intensive research, it has become obvious that, as with fruit, neglect rather than attention spoils a child. "I'd gotten so much pressure about spoiling the baby, even before she was born," says Judith, mother of three-year-old Kelsey. "But I felt differently inside. The information about the benefits of infant massage gave me permission to be the kind of mother I want to be and the research to back me up when I am contradicted." When we know why our caress is so important to our babies, we are more likely to follow our intuition, to relax, and to give way to our natural inclinations.

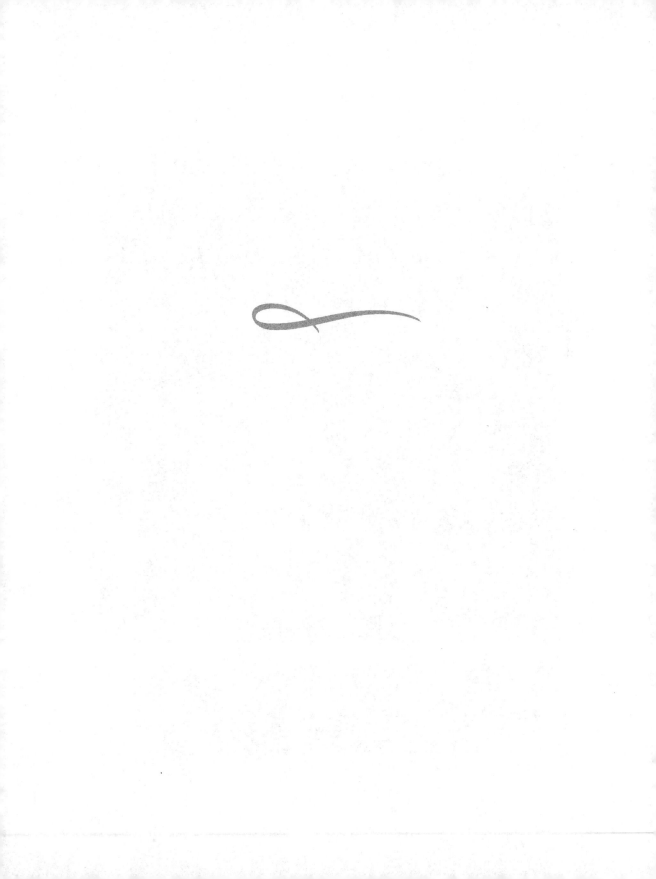

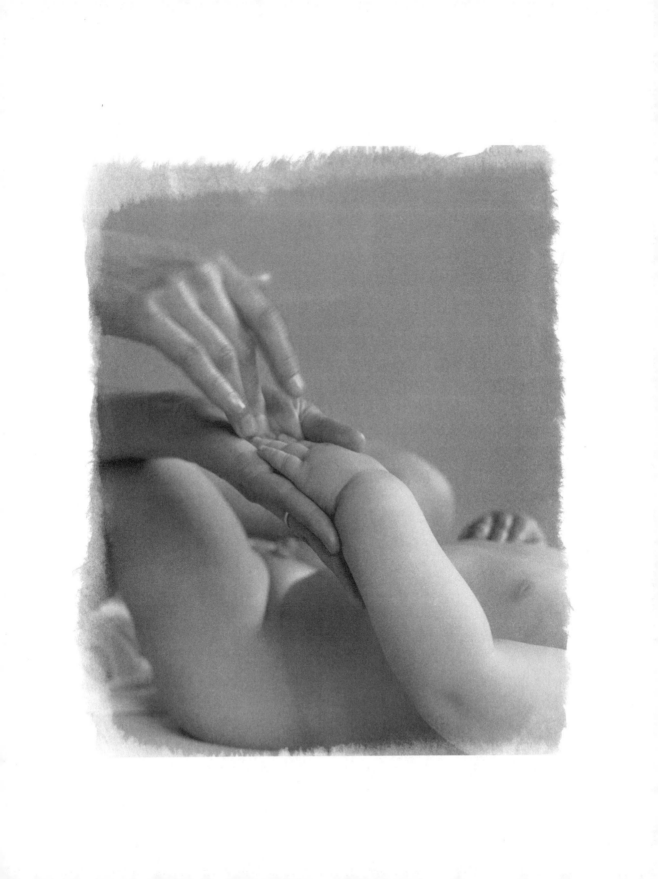

Chapter 2

Your Baby's Sensory World

Two little eyes to look around,
Two little ears to hear a sound,
One little nose to smell what's sweet,
One little mouth that likes to eat.

—TRADITIONAL NURSERY RHYME

A Baby's Senses Develop in Sequence

An infant's senses develop in sequence: first the proximity senses (those that need the nearness of some object to operate effectively), and then the distance senses (those that help the baby perceive things that are farther away). Of the proximity senses, the first and most important is touch.

Touch and Movement

The sense of touch has been detected in human embryos less than eight weeks old. Though the baby is less than an inch long and has no eyes or ears, her skin sensitivity is already highly developed. A fetus will pull away from an object that touches its face at eight weeks; by fourteen weeks, the infant can feel with most of his body. Her neural pathways for pain are fully developed at twenty-six weeks—indeed, premature infants born around this age have responded to painful stimuli. Medical scientists have recorded chemical stress reactions to potentially painful touches, such as that of a needle during amniocentesis, as early as twenty-three weeks, although they debate whether the baby can feel pain at this stage.

Nature begins the baby's massage long before she is born. First she rocks and floats, then slowly her world surrounds her ever more closely. The gentle caress of the womb becomes stronger, gradually becoming the contractions that rhythmically squeeze and push, providing massive stimulation to the infant's skin and organ systems. For babies birthed by Cesarean section, infant massage becomes an important way to stimulate the skin and organ systems.

Infants are accustomed to the tactile stimulation of constant movement, and they need the reestablishment of those rhythms after birth. In two studies, mothers in one group were asked to carry their infants not only during feeding or crying but for extra periods of time each day, in a soft front pack. These infants were compared with infants who were held and carried normally. At six weeks, the infants who received the extra touching and movement cried half as much as the others. Today kangaroo care is a common practice in hospital nurseries because of its beneficial effects on premature infants' physiological, social-emotional, and psychological health. Similarly, premature babies often receive massage as part of their care, now that Dr. Tiffany Field's studies have proven its remarkable impact on growth and development. More about this in Chapter 16.

Not only do newborns have a well-developed sense of touch, but this sense is vital to their survival. Many infants institutionalized in the United States in the early 1900s, and more recently babies in orphanages in Romania, died from what is now called failure to thrive. The cause of their death was not unsanitary conditions or lack of nutrition but the absence of human contact. Infants who survive their first six months but whose mothers fail to provide adequate touch fail to grow properly, researchers reported in 1994 in the *Journal of the American Academy of Child and Adolescent Psychiatry*.

Your baby's skin is her largest organ. More of her body is devoted to the sense of touch than to any other sense. Touching your baby, whether to feed, bathe, and change her or to cuddle, massage, and play with her, not only helps her grow but may also release endorphins, which make her happy, reduce pain, and heighten her other senses. According to the University of Pittsburgh Medical Center, infant massage may help strengthen your baby's immune system, improve her digestive and nervous systems, increase her muscle tone, and allow her to sleep more.

A May 2012 report from the *Cochrane Database of Systematic Reviews* states that newborns who had early skin-to-skin contact were warmer, cried less, interacted with their mothers more, and had greater levels of mother-infant attachment than babies who did not have this contact.

Taste and Smell

Other proximity senses are taste and smell, both of which are connected with touch and are significant to the newborn. A baby only five days old can differentiate her mother's smell and the taste of her milk from that of another mother. Infants, too, have special "chemical signatures" that their mothers are able to detect. Research shows that many mothers can pick out their infants' garments by scent alone after only two hours of exposure to their newborns.

Sight and Hearing

The distance senses—sight and hearing—can be very important to a baby's emotional attachment to his mother, an attachment that is essential to the development of a healthy parent-baby relationship. But the baby with a hearing and/or visual impairment will not suffer from lack of this bond if he has conscientious parents; the sense of touch and its impact upon maternal attachment are equally powerful. In fact, touch may be more dynamic, because it is the most significant and highly developed sense.

Even before birth, your baby can see. Before you know you are pregnant, the baby's optic nerve (the structure that transmits signals from the eye to the brain) has been formed. By six to seven months gestation, the baby's brain responds to light, and she can open and close her eyes, look up, down, and sideways. Your newborn is programmed to see you. Her eyes focus quite clearly at around seven to twelve inches—the distance at which your arms hold her comfortably. She is especially attracted to the high-contrast, bull's-eye shape of your eyes and nipples; this attraction enhances bonding through eye and skin contact and thus ensures her survival. In addition, the stimulation of gazing at these objects may enhance nerve myelination and physiological development.

In an article by Angela Ogunjimi for LiveStrong.com titled "Can a Baby Hear Outside Noises from Inside the Womb?" it is noted that a baby can hear her mom during pregnancy. The ears are complete by twenty-four weeks, when infants in utero can blink and are startled by stimulation. During the second trimester, babies begin to react to noises. Familiar voices may inspire a kick. The baby may startle at sudden sounds. After six months, the brain is developed enough for her to think. She may jump violently at a loud noise and be calmed by a lullaby. Our signature lullaby, "Ami Tomake Bhalobashi Baby," is sung with the massage and is available on CD to play in the background during pregnancy and beyond to soothe your baby.

In one experiment, babies were given four configurations of speech and sight from which to choose: the mother speaking normally, a stranger speaking normally, the mother appearing to speak in a stranger's voice, and a stranger appearing to speak in the mother's voice. The mother speaking normally was bliss. The babies looked less at a stranger speaking normally. But the mother-stranger mixes were intolerable, and the infants reacted with loud crying whenever they were presented to them. In another experiment, newborn infants were fitted with headphones through which they heard a voice telling a story. Whenever they sucked rapidly on a pacifier, they would hear their mother's voice; otherwise a stranger told the story. The infants learned how to cause their mother's voice to tell the story, and they preferred their mother's voice to any other.

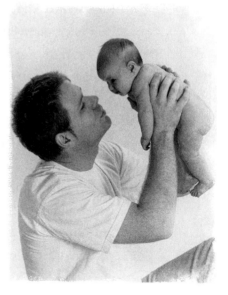

The beginnings of language learning can be seen in a baby's movement of her body in synchrony with her mother's speech patterns, intonations, and pauses. Computer studies analyzing movies of mothers and babies have revealed that each infant has a unique repertoire of body movements that synchronize with speech—a bodily response for every speech pattern. As the child grows older, these movements become microkinetic (discernible only through sophisticated instrumentation). At first the baby displays constant reflex movements, followed by the development of vocalization, then inflections, emotional content, and babbling. Finally words come, and ultimately these words have meaning of their own, no longer needing the reflex motor movements. But even a preschool child will move her foot when you ask her to say the word foot. There is still a trace of the parent's voice, internalized, saying "foot" as the infant body responds. The sounds a parent makes, including "parentese," or baby talk, and rhythmic songs and rhymes, appeal directly to the right hemisphere of the baby's brain, which is more highly developed than the left hemisphere at this stage.

The baby has been hearing his parents' voices from the time hearing developed in the womb, and the rhythms of speech even before that, through the reverberations of sounds that travel through the mother's bones. It is now believed that babies can begin to decipher language as early as six weeks of age. Other studies have shown that babies can differentiate different types of sentence structure and certain words that seem to go together, such as *the* before *dog*.

In 1997 studies by University of Washington neuroscientist Patricia

Kuhl showed that parents unconsciously exaggerate vowel sounds, which help babies develop a mastery of the phonetics of speech. For example, the word *bead,* she says, could easily be confused with *bed* or *bid.* But parents speak to their babies in "baby talk," saying, "Look at Mommy's beeeeeeds," in a high-pitched, singsong manner that stresses and exaggerates the vowels. Parents naturally provide the distinctions between vowel sounds that help their children learn to speak and, later, to read.

Kuhl found that six-month-olds categorize vowel sounds that are meaningful in their native language. She found parents' exaggeration of vowel sounds to be universal, in any language she studied. So it seems we are "programmed" to provide the auditory information that our babies need in order to begin to understand and speak their native tongue.

"I Love You!"

Later, when we begin doing infant massage, you will find that certain strokes can have rhymes or sounds associated with them, which accomplishes this same goal. While doing the stroke called I Love You on the baby's tummy, I encourage parents to elongate the vowels in a high-pitched voice. In every infant massage class I have taught or observed, the babies immediately attune to and are delighted with this particular stroke. Often,

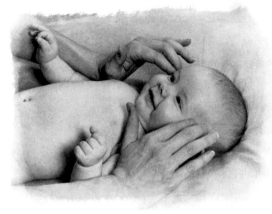

if some of the babies are fussing, all the parents in the room may simultaneously do the I Love You stroke, saying the words aloud with the sounds elongated. The fussing stops, and all the babies giggle and smile with rapt attention as the stroke is repeated. This stroke is the one most often requested by toddlers as well, who like to repeat the sounds with their parents as the stroke is done.

"Infant Stim"

While no one disputes that infants are drawn naturally to the types of stimulation they need for healthy development, researchers do disagree about the value of artificially stimulating an infant's distance senses. Advocates of early stimulation say that looking at stark black-and-white images (such as mobiles made of black-and-white bull's-eyes, checkerboards, and stripes), listening to recordings (including recordings of white noise—monotonous sounds such as vacuum cleaners and car engines), and other sensory stimuli may speed an infant's development and increase his intelligence, help an infant sleep, or soothe his colic.

Our great concern about our children's ability to compete on intelligence tests can drive us to accept programs that may or may not be valuable and that may in fact be detrimental to a child's long-term emotional and spiritual development. The makers of products for babies often imply that our children will not be able to compete for money and status in an increasingly competitive environment unless they are weaned to certain objects and ways of processing information as early as possible. Attaching the infant to material objects as "sensory stimulators" certainly benefits the companies that produce the products and the experts who promote them.

At the same time, parents who receive little or no cultural support for their role are often relieved of stress and guilt by these mechanical interventions. I am concerned about our slowly deteriorating intuitive abilities and confidence in ourselves. We may one day come to believe that material objects are actually better stimulators, more competent soothers, and more efficient brain-developers than we are, and that without these products our babies will be deprived. Instead of providing emotional nurturing, spiritual teaching, and exploration of the living world, we work harder and harder to provide our infants with the "necessary" objects of stimulation.

As researchers become more interested in the incredible array of benefits that massage can bring to infants, their interest has not gone unnoticed by profit-seekers. Many years ago I joked that if we wanted to make a lot of money, we could make a "baby massage device" that could be turned on and applied to the baby. The only problem would be that all of the benefits of infant massage would be forfeited.

To my immense shock and dismay, a company has actually made a "baby massager," similar to the Shiatsu massage devices so popular in malls (which usually end up in the closet, because nothing can ease tension like human touch). According to an article in *Digital Journal,* "It won't be long before exhausted parents everywhere can get much needed relief with a groundbreaking infant massaging device." This device is being hailed as the answer to parents' stress. The device "naturally" soothes a crying baby by simulating the mother's touch. Called "unique and innovative," the invention "also features quick clips for one-handed fastening to baby's clothing; soft, relaxing music; and a playback of the mother's voice, as well as safety features such as an auto shut-off if baby rolls on top of it."

Generally, nothing much bothers me these days. But when I read these articles and saw photos of the device, I was floored. The purposes of infant massage include making eye-to-eye contact, hearing a parent's voice, smelling the parent's unique scent, and experiencing skin-to-skin touch, all important in the bonding of babies with their parents. Massage also helps develop gastrointestinal, circulatory, and respiratory functions. The massage taught by the International Association of Infant Massage emphasizes emotional and spiritual bonding between baby and parent; each stroke is different and has its own function. Stroke sequences to help babies relax and pass painful gas are included. The massage we teach takes from fifteen minutes to half an hour—hardly an addition to a parent's stress. In fact, it has been found that massaging the baby relaxes and soothes the parent as well. Regular infant massage relaxes, soothes, bonds, and helps eliminate problems such as colic. No device could possibly replace a loving parent's hands delivering a real massage.

When I saw this device, I thought, "Here we go—soon we'll have mechanical devices we can put our babies into, so we won't have to touch them or make time for soothing them at all." It is shocking to me that the writers of these articles hail the device as "groundbreaking" and love its "sleek, futuristic design." There are no studies proving that this type of device has any benefits at all, much less the benefits of a parent delivering a massage skin to skin, responding to the baby's cues, and looking into the baby's eyes with love, singing or talking to the baby all the while. But I worry that many unknowing parents will buy it, thinking it will benefit their babies.

Developmental psychologists today agree that infants are natural learners and will extract from a warm, loving environment whatever information they need. The basic security provided by a strong parent-infant bond enables babies to reach out to their world and to develop to their full capacity physically, mentally, and spiritually. Infant massage provides a wealth of fascinating sensory experiences. Your eyes, your hairline, your smile, your scent, and the sound of your voice telling a story or singing a lullaby provide not only the interesting contrast your baby looks for but also warm, loving feedback. It not only speeds the myelination of her nerves but lets her know she has come into a living, breathing world. There is no sweeter music than the sound of a mother singing; there will never be a toy that can tell a story the way a real live daddy can. No one can invent a substitute for a parent's loving touch. No vestibular stimulation device can compare with being rocked and carried in loving arms. And as for white noise, nothing can surpass the sounds of breath and heart in synchrony.

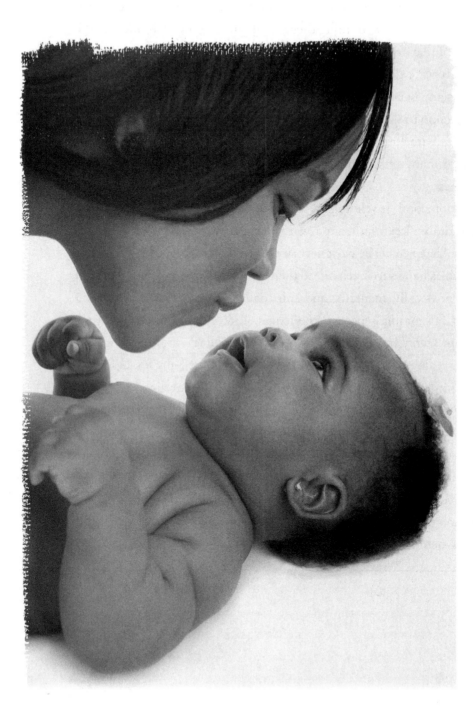

Chapter 3

The Importance of Skin Stimulation

Throw away gadgets. Discard
expert opinions. Forget the toys
to stimulate intelligence. Don't buy
devices to simulate what is real.

Return to the real. Connect with
your children heart to heart.
Let them gaze at you, at trees
and water and sky. Let them feel
their pain. Feel it with them.

Touch them with your hands,
your eyes, and your heart.
Let them bond with the living,
breathing world. Let them feel
their feelings and teach them
their names.

Return to the uncarved simplicity.

—VIMALA MCCLURE,
THE TAO OF MOTHERHOOD

Skin Stimulation Is Important for Mammals

Skin sensitivity is the earliest-developed and most fundamental function of the body. Nurturing stimulation of the skin is, in fact, essential for adequate organic and psychological development, both for animals and for human beings. When asked what he thought of infant massage, anthropologist Ashley Montagu commented, "People don't realize that communication for a baby, the first communications it receives and the first language of its development, is through the skin. If only most people had realized this they would have all along given babies the kind of skin stimulation they require."

Behaviorally, mammals tend to fall into "cache" and "carry" types. The caching species leave their young for long periods while the mother gathers food. The infants must remain silent during those times so as not to attract predators, so they do not cry. For the same reason, they do not urinate unless stimulated by the mother. In addition, the young have internal mechanisms that control their body temperature. The mother's milk is extremely high in protein and fat, and the infants suckle at a very fast rate.

In contrast, the carrying species maintain continuous contact with their infants and feed often. The babies suckle slowly, urinate often, cry when distressed or out of contact with the parent, and need the parent to keep them warm. The mother's milk content is low in protein and fat, so infants need to suckle often. Humans are designed like the carrying species; in fact, human milk is identical in protein and fat content to that of the anthropoid apes, which are carrying species. Our infants need to be in close physical contact with us as much as possible.

No Colicky Kittens!

Physically, massage acts in much the same way in humans as licking does in animals. Animals lick their young and maintain close skin contact. Animal babies that are not licked, caressed, and permitted to cling in infancy grow up scrawny and more vulnerable to stress. They tend to fight with one another and to abuse and neglect their own young. Licking serves to stimulate the physiological systems and to bond the young with the mother. A mother cat spends more than 50 percent of her time licking her babies—and you will never see a colicky kitten! Without the kind of stimulation that helps their gastrointestinal system begin to function properly, newborn kittens die.

Scientists have seen behavior and responses in animals that parallel the growth and development of our own young, and these parallels are truly fascinating. In animals, the genitourinary tract will not function without the stimulation of frequent licking. Even the number of times a mother licks her young and the amount of time spent in each area are genetically determined.

Animals Benefit with Higher Immunity

When the infant mammal receives early skin stimulation, there is a highly beneficial influence on the immunological system. In one experiment, rats that were gently handled in infancy had a higher serum antibody standard in every case. More simply stated, these animals had a much greater ability to resist disease.

Equally important for our purposes was the behavior of these gentled rats. As Ashley Montagu wrote in *Touching:*

When handled, the gentled animals were relaxed and yielding. They were not easily frightened. . . . The researcher who had raised them . . . did so under conditions in which they were frequently handled, stroked, and had kindly sounds uttered to them, and they responded with fearlessness, friendliness, and a complete lack of neuromuscular tension or irritability. The exact opposite was true of the ungentled rats, who had received no attention whatever from human beings . . . these animals were frightened and bewildered, anxious and tense.

Among other important findings, rats that were gently handled for three weeks after weaning showed a faster weight gain than other rats under the same conditions, and those that were handled gently were physically much more resistant to the harmful effects of stress and deprivation.

In one study, rats with their thyroid and parathyroid glands (endocrine glands that regulate the immune system) removed responded remarkably to massage. In the experimental group, the rats were gently massaged and spoken to several times a day. They were relaxed, yielding, and not easily frightened, and their nervous systems remained stable. The control rats, which did not receive this type of care, were nervous, fearful, irritable, and enraged; they died within forty-eight hours. Another study with rats showed a higher immunity to disease, faster weight gain, and better neurological development among those that had been gently stroked in infancy.

Moving up the animal scale, dogs, horses, cows, dolphins, and many other animals have also shown remarkable differences when lovingly handled in infancy. The touch of the human hand improved the function of virtually all of the sustaining systems (respiratory, circulatory, digestive, eliminative, nervous, and endocrine) and increased "touchability," gentleness, friendliness, and fearlessness. Writes Ashley Montagu: "The more we learn about the effects of cutaneous [skin] stimulation, the more pervasively significant for healthy development do we find it to be."

Harry Harlow's famous monkey experiments were the first to show that for infants, contact comfort is even more important than food. Infant monkeys, given the choice of a wire mother figure that provided food, or a soft terry-cloth figure that did not provide food, chose the terry-cloth mother figure. Human infants with failure-to-thrive syndrome exhibit the same type of behavior: though given all the food they need, they continue to deteriorate if they receive no intervention that involves emotional nurturing, contact comfort, and care.

In nearly every bird and mammal studied, close physical contact has been found to be essential both to the infant's healthy survival and to the mother's ability to nurture. In the previously mentioned studies with rats, if pregnant females were restrained from licking themselves (a form of self-massage), their mothering activities were substantially diminished. Additionally, when pregnant female animals were gently stroked every day, their offspring showed higher weight gain and reduced excitability, and the mothers showed greater interest in their offspring, with a more abundant and richer milk supply.

Skin Stimulation Is Important for Human Babies

Evidence supports the same conclusions for humans. Touching and handling her baby assists the new mother in milk production by helping stimulate secretion of prolactin, the "mothering hormone." The process begun at the embryonic stage thus continues, allowing a natural unfolding of the baby's potential within the safe and loving arms of his mother.

Nurturing stimulation of the skin—handling, cuddling, rocking, and massage—increases cardiac functions of the human infant. Massage stimulates the respiratory, circulatory, and gastrointestinal systems—benefits especially appreciated by the "colicky" baby and his parents.

A baby's first experience with the surrounding environment occurs through touch, developing prenatally as early as sixteen weeks. Nature begins the massage before the baby is born. As opposed to the extremely short labors of most other animals, it has been suggested that a human mother's extended labor helps make up for the lack of postpartum licking performed by other mammal mothers. For the human infant, the contractions of labor provide some of the same type of preparation for the functioning of his internal systems as early licking of the newborn does for other mammals.

Touch impacts short-term development during infancy and early childhood, and it has long-term effects as well. Through this contact, newborns are able to learn about their world, bond with their parents, and communicate their needs and wants. Eighty percent of a baby's communication is expressed through body movement. When parents engage in appropriate touch, young children have an improved chance to successfully develop socially, emotionally, and intellectually.

Infants who experience more physical contact with parents demonstrate increased mental development in the first six months of life compared to young children who receive limited physical interaction. This improved cognitive development has been shown to last even after eight years, illustrating the importance of positive interactions. Infants who receive above-average levels of affection from their parents are shown to be less likely to be hostile, anxious, or emotionally distressed as adults.

Studies with premature babies using techniques similar to those taught in this book have demonstrated that daily massage is of tremendous benefit. Research projects at the University of Miami Medical Center, headed up by the Touch Research Institute's founder, Dr. Tiffany Field, have shown remarkable results. In one study, twenty premature babies were massaged three times a day for fifteen minutes each time. They averaged 47 percent greater weight gain per day, were more active and alert, and showed more mature neurological development than infants who did not receive massage. In addition, their hospital stay averaged six days less. After many years of study and observation, the International Association of Infant Massage has established guidelines for using massage and holding techniques with premature babies. We'll look more closely at this in Chapter 16.

Dallas psychologist Ruth Rice conducted a study with thirty premature babies after they had left the hospital. She divided them into two groups. The mothers in the control group were instructed in usual newborn care, while those in the experimental group were taught a daily massage and rocking regime. At four months of age, the babies who had been massaged were ahead in both neurological development and weight gain.

The natural sensory stimulation of massage speeds myelination of the brain and the nervous system. The myelin sheath is a fatty covering around each nerve, like insulation around electrical wire. It protects the nervous system and speeds the transmission of impulses from the brain to the rest of the body. The process of coating the nerves is not complete at birth, but skin stimulation hastens the process, thus enhancing rapid neural-cell firing and improving brain-body communication.

In 1978 transcutaneous oxygen monitoring was developed, which enabled physicians to measure oxygen tension in the body through an electrode on the skin. It was discovered that hospitalized infants experienced tremendous upheavals in oxygen levels when subjected to stress. Touch Relaxation, holding techniques, and massage (Chapters 9, 12, and 13) have been found to mitigate these fluctuations, and these methods are being used in hospitals routinely now to help infants maintain a steady state through the stresses of diaper changes, heel sticks, and other intrusions.

New research demonstrates similar results every day, confirming what age-old tradition has told us: infants need loving touch. Lawrence Schachner, M.D., a professor in the Department of Dermatology and Cutaneous Surgery at the University of Miami Miller School of Medicine, advises that touch can benefit babies with skin disorders such as eczema. "It may furthermore improve parent-baby interaction," he says. Dr. Tiffany Field concurs. She notes that loving touch triggers physiological changes that help infants grow and develop, stimulating nerves in the brain that facilitate food absorption and lowering stress hormone levels, resulting in improved immune system functioning. A report by the Families and Work Institute states that the vast majority of connections between brain cells are formed during the first three years of life. The report concludes that loving interaction such as massage can directly affect a child's emotional development and ability to handle stress as an adult.

Loving skin contact and massage benefit mothers and fathers as well.

In addition, research has shown that mothers whose pregnancies were filled with chronic stress often have babies who cry more and for longer periods than those whose pregnancies were peaceful and supported.

Men who make the effort to bond with their infants by giving the mother loving massages, talking and singing to the baby, feeling its movements in their partner's belly, attending classes with their partner, and reading up on infant development and psychology tend to be more attentive and accomplished fathers.

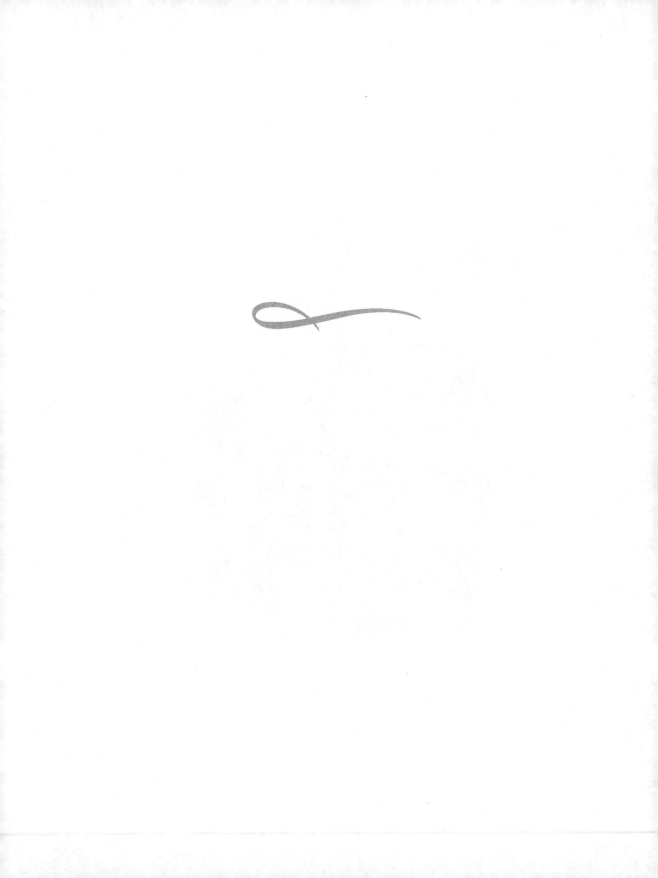

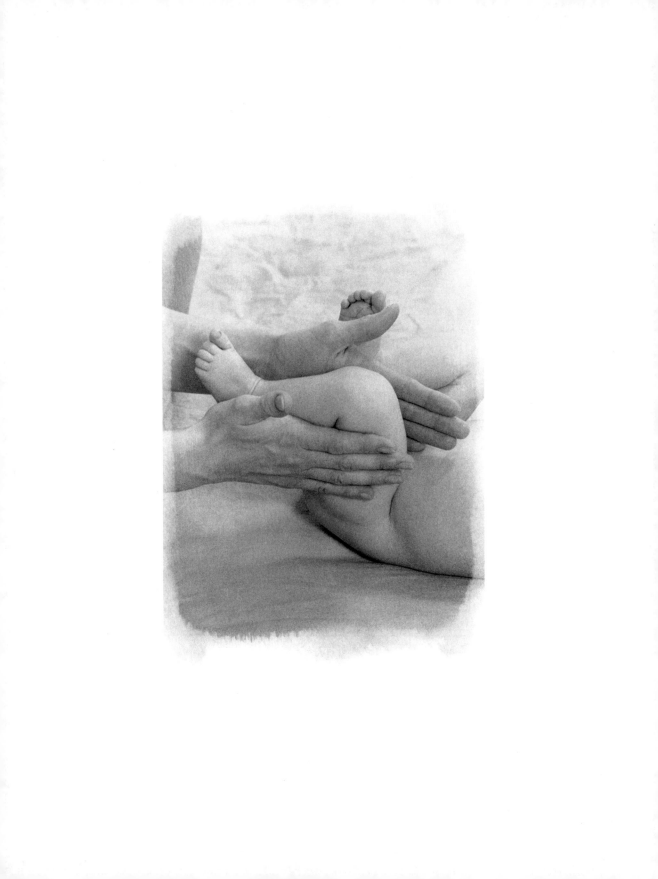

Chapter 4

Stress and Relaxation

First-time mothers read all the books
and cling to theories and gadgets.

Fifth-time mothers have taken it all in
and let it sink into the unconscious.
Equipment has worn out and the child
is given wooden spoons and the easy
company of present-focused people.
The youngest child is usually the most
relaxed!

—VIMALA MCCLURE,
THE TAO OF MOTHERHOOD

A Balance

In our great-great-grandmothers' day, when a baby developed a fever, the outcome was uncertain. Each century's children have been plagued with some debilitating disease. Though many contagions have been eliminated through improved environmental conditions and medicine, our century is characterized by a more subtle and insidious malady—stress.

Stress can begin to affect a baby even before he is born. The levels of stress hormones that are constantly present in a woman's bloodstream directly affect her unborn infant, crossing the placenta to enter his own bloodstream. Studies have shown that prolonged tension and anxiety can hamper a pregnant woman's ability to absorb nourishment. Her baby may be of low birth weight, hyperactive, and irritable.

If we understand that our experiences and reactions influence our own biochemistry by sending life-enhancing or fear-producing chemicals throughout our bodies, it is not difficult to understand that these chemicals are also sent through our unborn baby's body. Her cells receive this "information" and program her structure accordingly. Thus, even before birth, a baby can unconsciously perceive the world as a place of anxiety and stress, something to fight or to be victimized by, or as a place of safety and love, something to enjoy and fully experience. This is not to say all is lost if life circumstances are less than perfect. Infant massage is one tool we have to help reshape our child's interpretations of the world, to release her pain, grief, and fear, and to open her up to love and joy. As we evolve to be more conscious beings, we understand more deeply how important our mind states are, both to our own health and longevity and to our children's health, longevity, intelligence, and ability to experience and give love and joy.

Babies born centuries ago in more primitive cultures had the advantage of extended families, natural environments, and relatively little change. Our children, born into a rapidly advancing technological world, must effectively handle stress if they are to survive and prosper. Thus we must give them every opportunity, from conception on, to learn positive, adaptive responses to stress and to believe in their own power and adaptability.

We certainly cannot eliminate stress, nor would we wish to, for in the proper doses it is an essential component in the growth of intelligence. Let's see how this works. In times of stress, the pituitary gland produces a hormone called ACTH (adrenocorticotropic hormone), which activates the adrenal steroids, mobilizing the body and brain to deal with an unknown or unpredictable emergency. In experiments with laboratory animals, this hormone has been found to stimulate the production of many new proteins in the liver and brain—proteins that are instrumental in both learning and memory. When animals are given ACTH, their brains grow millions of new connecting links between the neurons (thinking cells). These links enable the brain to process information.

The stress of meeting unknown situations and converting them into what is known and predictable is essential for our babies' brain development. But stress is only part of the cycle that enhances learning. Without its equally important opposite, relaxation, stress can lead to overstimulation, exhaustion, and shock. When stress piles upon stress without the relief of an equal portion of relaxation, the body begins to shut out all sensory intake and the learning process is completely blocked. As neuroscientist Bruce Lipton described, in a competition between protection-related biological behavior and growth-promoting biological behavior, the protection-related behavior wins out, thus preventing growth or learning.

How does this apply to infant massage? First, massage is one way we can provide our children with relaxing, joyful experiences. Through the use of conditioned-response techniques similar to those developed for childbirth by Lamaze and others (see the section on Touch Relaxation in Chapter 9), we can teach our babies how to relax their bodies in response to stress. The ability to relax consciously is a tremendous advantage in coping with the pressures of growing up in modern society. If acquired early in life, the relaxation response can become as much a part of our children's natural system as the antibodies that protect them from disease.

Stress is a natural part of an infant's life, but often our babies are not able to benefit from it as much as they could. Our fast-paced society overloads them with input, but it is unacceptable for them to cry to release tension. This double bind leads to many frustrated babies with a lot of pent-up tension and anxiety.

Massage helps babies practice handling input and responding to it with relaxation. Watch an experienced mother massaging her baby. You will see both stress and relaxation in the rhythmic strokes and in the baby's reactions. The infant experiences all kinds of new sensations, feelings, odors, sounds, and sights. The rumbles of his tummy, the warm sensation of increased circulation, the movement of air on his bare skin—all are mildly stressful. The pleasant tone of his mother's voice, her smile, and her touch are relaxing and relieve the discomfort of encountering these new sensations. She reassures him that the world outside the womb is, as Dr. Frédérick Leboyer says, "still alive, and warm, and beating, and friendly."

A daily massage raises an infant's stimulation threshold. Babies who have difficulty handling stimulation gradually build tolerance. High-need babies begin to learn to regulate the manner in which they respond to stressful experiences, which reduces the level of tension they develop throughout the day. Colicky babies are calmed and able to relax their bodies so that tension doesn't escalate their discomfort. A regular massage provides our babies with an early stress management program that will be valuable to them in years to come.

Into Adulthood

Psychologists study the types of attachments we form in our infancy as predictors of the types of relationships we will have as adults. People whose infancy was secure, who were held and listened to, who had good eye contact with their parents, and who were generally cherished tend to have healthier relationships with others. Getting close to others is easy, and there's no problem with interdependency (the ability to depend on and be depended on, appropriately). They have happy, trusting relationships; their romances last the longest and end in divorce the least often of groups studied. On the other hand, babies whose attachment bonds are insecure or anxious are later less sympathetic to others and less effective in getting support and help from other people. Their relationships lack trust and intimacy; jealousy, commitment problems, and fears undermine friendships as well as marriages. People whose bonds are constantly broken in infancy have a much greater risk of becoming sociopathic criminals in their adulthood, unless they receive serious intervention at an early age.

The connection between the emotional brain and the rational brain is important as well. A child can experience feelings of fear or rage, even excessive excitement, and may not be able to handle the emotions, not knowing how to regulate them appropriately. An overstimulated child throwing a tantrum without a caring parental response may well become an out-of-control, angry adult.

The bonds of trust and love, along with the lessons of compassion, warmth, openness, and respect that are inherent in the massage routine, will be carried by your child into adulthood. Especially if your parenting practices reflect the same values of infant massage, your child will be more likely to respond to others with empathy and warmth, to respond to social problems with compassion and altruism, and to experience life as a joyful adventure in which he has the opportunity to love and be loved—to help others and extend himself in genuine service to humanity.

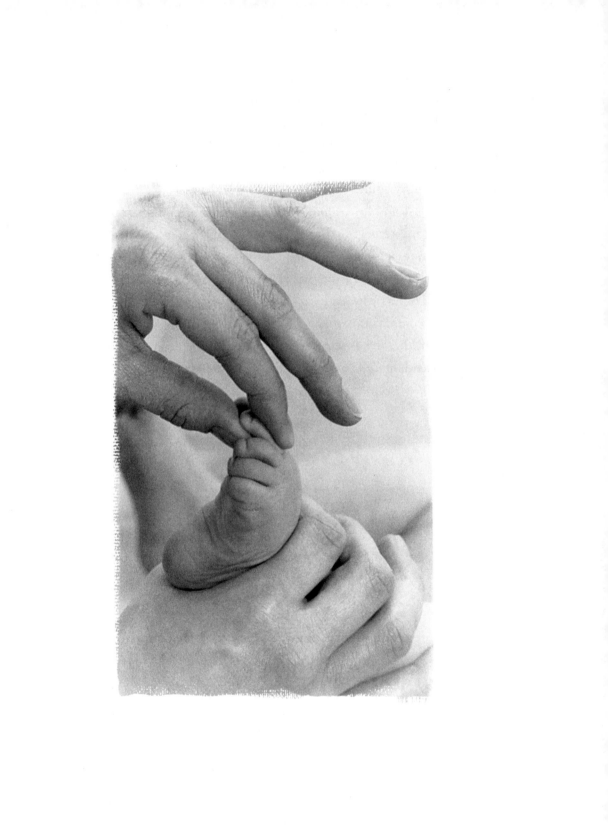

Chapter 5

Bonding, Attachment, and Infant Massage

Baby, I lie and gaze on thee
All other things forgot—
In dreams the things of earth pass by
But awake I heed them not.
I hear thy soft breath come and go,
Thy breath so lately given,
And watch the blue unconscious eyes
Whose light is pure from heaven.
—ANONYMOUS, NINETEENTH CENTURY

The Profound Impact of Bonding

What Is Bonding?

Bonding is a basic phenomenon that occurs throughout the universe. In terms of physics, it is established within the energy field from which particles arise. Two particles of energy brought into proximity spin and polarize in an interconnected way, even when separated. Two living cells of a human heart brought into proximity begin to beat together. Throughout the animal kingdom and in human life as well, affectionate and tactile bonds between mother and young ensure healthy interaction and development for time to come. Proximity between parent and infant, via sensory experiences and loving interactions, brings them into an important synchrony with each other. Bonding is the process by which the parent forms an attachment to the infant.

In animals, the crucial period for bonding is usually a matter of minutes or hours after birth. The mother bonds with her infant through licking and touching, which in turn help the infant to physically adjust to extrauterine life. If mother and infant are separated during this time and then are subsequently reunited, the mother will often reject or neglect her young. As a result, the newborn may die for lack of mother's stimulation, even if fed by other means.

In studies paralleling animal behavior, John Kennell and Marshall Klaus, among others, have revealed that there is also a sensitive period for bonding in humans; however, the crucial period seems less rigidly defined. The attachment process continues for months and even years after childbirth.

Dramatic evidence in the Kennell and Klaus studies correlates the lack of early bonding with later child abuse, neglect, and failure-to-thrive syndrome. Mothers who are separated from their infants during the newborn period are often more hesitant and clumsy in learning basic mothering tasks.

Unattached and anxiously attached infants can grow up to exhibit a range of disorders, from difficulty in forming and maintaining relationships at one end of the spectrum all the way to sociopathic criminal behavior at the other. Anxiously attached means that a baby is not consistently responded to with love by her caregivers, so the baby cannot relax and depend on her needs being met and the world being a good and friendly place to be. Such children are fearful of the world and have a difficult time trusting and opening up to others, and they often have buried anger that can come out inappropriately later in life. Solid, loving attachments are hard for them to make because, as anxiously attached babies, they did not learn how to trust.

Clinical data is beginning to show us what many mothers all over the world have known for generations—that loving, touching, nurturing contact between parent and infant has a very real impact upon the child's subsequent development. In short, the attachment of a parent to her/his newborn is not merely sweet sentimentality—it is a demonstrated biological necessity.

Human Babies Cannot Initiate Bonding

Unlike the clinging monkey, the human infant has no physical means of initiating contact with his mother and thus getting his needs fulfilled. His life depends upon the strength of his parents' emotional attachment to him. Where there is early and extended mother-baby contact, studies show impressively positive results. Mothers who bonded with their babies in the first hours and days of life later showed greater closeness to their babies, exhibited much more soothing behavior, maintained more eye contact, and touched their babies more often. Early-contact mothers were more successful in breastfeeding, they spent more time looking at their infants during feeding, and their babies' weight gain was greater. These children had significantly higher IQ scores on the Stanford–Binet test at age three than children who had been separated from their mothers.

Infant Day Care

Experts who have studied the effects of day care on babies under one year of age sounded the alarm as early as 1985, when many studies began to support the conclusion that poor-quality day care, poor-quality home care, and too-early day care can cause long-term stresses and possible damage to important parent-infant bonds.

Many years later we are alarmed at the number of children who have little or no conscience about using violence as a way to gain status, peer acceptance, and relief from fears and frustrations. Though many factors contribute to this phenomenon, including the assault of inappropriate media, more tolerance for violence in our culture as a whole, the disintegration of extended family bonds, and the financial pressures that put unreasonable strain on every family, some experts suggest that breaks in the attachment process can go deep into an infant's psychology, engendering rage that finally expresses itself by hurting another being. Separation from the primary parent too early in life can threaten bonds and wreak havoc on the child's later life and family harmony. Children whose bonding has been anxious or inadequate or whose family is unable to exert influence and boundaries on behavior often grow up with serious psychosocial problems that are difficult to address and heal.

Many new parents have little choice with regard to their contribution to the family income, making day care a significant issue for every new family. So the information here is not meant to engender guilt in working parents. It is not day care versus stay-at-home parenting that is important to evaluate, though that is a decision to be made carefully. I believe the most important aspect of this subject is the quality of care the baby receives, regardless of who delivers it, and the quality of the environment at home when the baby returns. That said, I still believe that parents are a young infant's best caregivers because this is the time when the most important bonds of attachment form, which impact for life a baby's psychology and behavior and thus the way she is responded to by peers and culture.

Dr. Ken Magid emphasizes the dangers of too-early day care in his book *High Risk: Children Without a Conscience*. "After reviewing all the literature, it is my opinion that no child should be left for any significant period of time during the first year of life," he says. "Parents of small infants must proceed with extreme caution when they are considering turning care of their baby over to someone else, whether it be a babysitter or relative. These are the most important moments of your baby's life."

In research done by the National Institute on Child Health and Development in 1996, 1,300 families were followed as the children grew from infancy to age seven; they were observed both in day care settings and at home. The study found that infants in low-quality day care or infants who had several different caregivers in day care were more likely to develop anxious or insecure attachments if their mothers were also unresponsive to their needs. So it is not necessarily the amount of time an infant is in day care but the quality of interaction in the family, the quality of environment in the day care, and the quality of interaction with day care providers (preferably as few as possible) that affect whether an infant can develop healthy bonds. The lack of such interaction, however, is just as powerful. Infants in lower-quality institutional day care tend to receive minimal touch, which is associated with long-lasting cognitive delays in the future. Touch deprivation is additionally associated with increased aggression, pointing to the emotional and behavioral impact of contact during early childhood.

Studies also show that high-quality day care can prevent the drop in IQ that happens between twelve and thirty months of age in babies kept in home-reared, low-income environments. It seems that whether an infant is in day care is not the most important issue. A stressful environment in which an infant is not given the love, affection, and relaxed attention he needs seems to be the highest risk factor for developing an attachment disorder. Thus, even if a parent stays home to care for a baby, if the loss of income and self-esteem puts the parent under undue stress, this in itself will affect the baby adversely, more so than if the baby was in a high-quality day care situation with one or two consistent, loving caregivers and the parents were happy at home and could provide the baby with love, affection, play, and focused attention outside of work.

Parents who simply cannot take time off from work to care for their newborn infants get little help from our culture in providing substitute care that is of acceptable quality. They must suffer the anguish of separation from their infants, the feelings of guilt that result, and worries about the adequacy of the care they have chosen. Often these feelings in themselves serve to distance parents from their infants and further deteriorate bonds that should be strengthened.

Massage for a Baby in Day Care

A daily massage can be of tremendous help in maintaining and strengthening affectionate bonds between parents and an infant in day care. Taking a half hour for reconnecting through massage after work can help a parent refocus on home life and help an infant to feel secure and supported.

"Our baby loves his massage and typically smiles and coos throughout," says Barbara, mother of six-month-old John. "Since both my husband and I work outside the home, the massage is a way to tune out work and reconnect with John and each other after a stressful day. We are convinced that our baby is happy and relaxed because of the time we spend massaging him."

Other working parents find that their infants often spend part of the massage time fussing. One mother told me she thought her baby liked the day care provider more than her, because he always cried hard the first hour or so at home and fussed through the first part of his massage, whereas he seemed very happy in day care. Often she just stopped massaging him and let him cry himself to sleep; she felt frustrated and inadequate as a parent. Her view of the situation changed when I suggested that his crying indicated just the opposite: he saved his expression of stress until he was with her, the safest environment in which he could release pent-up tension from all the day's stimulation. Considering his crying this way, she could help him release his stress by empathizing with him through her voice and body language, and continuing the massage using holding techniques and stopping for comfort breaks. Within a few weeks, her baby cried less and less. Eventually they bonded closely, and she could massage him after work feeling competent, loving, and secure in the knowledge that she was a good mother and her baby felt safe with her above all others. He settled into the massage and began to enjoy it, cooing and gazing at his mother, relaxing into the rhythmic strokes and the sound of her voice soothing him.

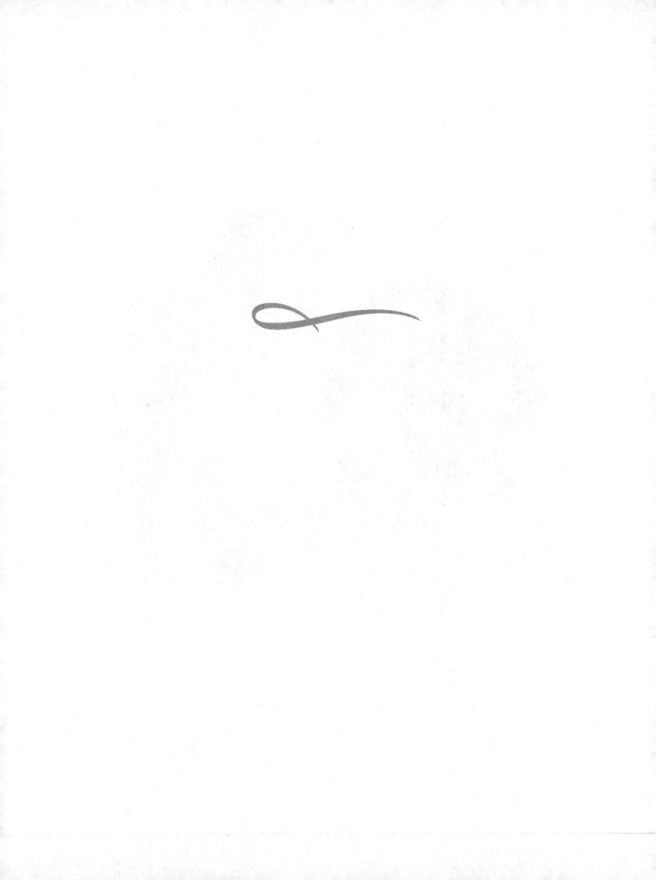

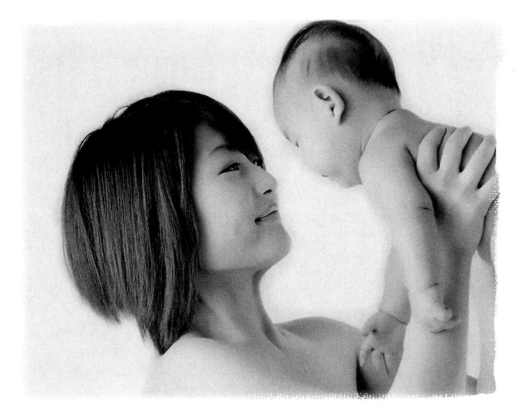

Chapter 6

The Elements of Bonding

*There is nothing more receptive
and flowing than water,
yet there is nothing better
for polishing stone.*

*A mother's nature is paradox.
Your strength is in gentleness.
Your authority is in receptivity.
Your power is in letting go.*

—VIMALA MCCLURE,
THE TAO OF MOTHERHOOD

Each Element Contained in Infant Massage

The important elements that help form the bond between parent and infant include eye contact, skin contact, vocalization, the baby's responses to the parent, the activation of maternal and paternal hormones by contact with the baby, temperature regulation, and the immunizing bacteria and antibodies transferred to the baby by close contact with the parents.

While all of these elements come into play during the massage routine, the vital elements that strengthen bonds are:

Skin-to-skin contact

Prolonged and steady eye-to-eye contact

The soothing, high-pitched sounds of a parent's voice

The odor of mother-to-baby and baby-to-mother

Engagement (talking, gaze-shifting, singing)

Infant massage, which serves as communication between parent and infant, helps cement the bond. The baby learns to enjoy the wonderful comfort and security of loving and being loved. He acquires knowledge about his own body, as his parent shows him how to relax a tense arm or back, or helps him release some painful gas.

For parents as well, massaging their infant is a lesson in relaxation and centering. The massage is a perfect way for a parent to practice mindfulness—a mental state achieved by focusing one's awareness on the present moment while calmly acknowledging and accepting one's feelings, thoughts, and bodily sensations.

At one time or another, every parent has felt tense and nervous, and in spite of their best efforts, baby begins to fuss and cry. Since babies are such incredibly sensitive little beings, it is important that parents make massage time a period of relaxation for themselves as well. A simple twenty-minute massage can provide a welcome respite from and transition out of the fussy-baby/tense-parent cycle.

Eye Contact

Eye contact is one of the most powerful communication systems we have. Between parent and infant, it is a vital connecting link. Parents seem compelled to get into a face-to-face position with their newborns and to gaze into their eyes. New parents croon to their babies, "Come on, now—open your eyes. Are you going to look at me?" Delighted exclamations follow when the infant makes eye contact. Parents report that they first feel very close to their babies when eye contact is made. The baby's visual system is biologically programmed to search out the contrasts in the bull's-eye shape of the parent's eyes and nipples. Maternal hormones darken the areola during pregnancy, perhaps to help attract the baby's gaze. Experts speculate that eye contact may be a powerful cue to the infant's physiological system: the message received by the brain allows it to shut down the production of stress hormones initiated during childbirth. During a massage, the infant is positioned face-to-face with the parent, and the quality of interaction provides a lot of positive feedback, via eye contact, for parent and baby, continually reinforcing the message "It is okay to relax now."

Skin Contact

Mothers seem to instinctively stroke their babies after birth, bringing myelination to the nerves and awakening the senses. Touch is a powerful element in human bonding. People in love, children forming friendships, and even people who have acquired a new pet will spend extra time in close contact until the bond is secure. Animals raised without touch grow up to be antisocial and aggressive, and they tend to abuse and neglect their own young. Neurologist Richard Restak, author of *The Infant Mind,* comments on the importance of touch:

The infant turns toward the mother. How will she respond? Will she touch him? Will she turn away? How simple the situation, how seemingly devoid of content and importance. But we are deceived by the simplicity of this exchange which takes place within seconds but endures for decades. The mother turns toward her infant and touches him. Neither party speaks. Who could ever have guessed that simply touching another human being could be so important.

Touch can benefit both mothers and infants alike, forming a bond between parent and child. Infants of depressed mothers who massage their infants show improvement in growth and development while the mothers' depression levels decrease. Physical contact can also lower levels of cortisol, a stress hormone, for both mothers and babies, leading to improved immune system functioning. By continually providing nurturing touch, parents can help facilitate enhanced social, emotional, and physical development in their children at a young age.

In hospitals in Western cultures, babies are routinely separated from their mothers, particularly when infants are premature or medically at risk, even though research has shown the advantages of maternal touch for all newborns. This separation is relatively new among humans, and humans are the only mammals who now separate their newborns from mothers. A study in the journal *Biological Psychiatry* monitored the difference between newborns' heart rates, digestions, and respiratory rates when in skin-to-skin contact with their mothers and when sleeping in a bassinet beside their mothers' beds. The editor of the journal commented on the study's findings: "This paper highlights the profound impact of maternal separation on the infant. We knew that this was stressful, but the current study suggests that this is a major stressor for the infant."

If you want to create a transition environment for your baby that imitates aspects of the experience in utero, you may want to get a baby pack or sling that keeps your infant close to your body so she can hear your heartbeat. Some pastel organza material, draped over the cradle, can soften the light. Putting a warm cap on her head when going outdoors will prevent heat from escaping through her head. A baby monitor can help alert you to your baby's sounds if you are in another room. Other aids include a heartbeat simulator for the baby's cradle and setting the volume low on your stereo, television, and phone.

Cosleeping

Some parents want to try family cosleeping, which is a much-debated practice in Westernized countries. My family practiced cosleeping until my youngest was around five years old. The tales of accidental suffocation by "overlying" are just that: tales. Dr. James J. McKenna, director of the Mother-Baby Behavioral Sleep Laboratory at University of Notre Dame, says, "It is a curious fact that in Western societies the practice of mothers, fathers, and infants sleeping together came to be thought of as strange, unhealthy, and dangerous. Western parents are taught that cosleeping will make the infant too dependent on them, or risk accidental suffocation. Such views are not supported by human experience worldwide." Research has suggested that many mothers who have been diagnosed as having postpartum depression are actually suffering extreme fatigue from waking to their babies at night.

Research was done by McKenna and his colleagues, who invited thirty-five mother-baby pairs into a sleep research laboratory and monitored their sleep patterns overnight as they slept together or in separate rooms. They found that not only did cosleeping pairs get into the same sleep cycles, but that babies who coslept experienced more frequent arousals, triggered by the mother's movements, and spent less time in deep sleep.

Having done research on sudden infant death syndrome (SIDS), Professor McKenna believes that these low-level arousals, which did not actually awaken either partner, give the baby practice in arousing itself. This may lessen a baby's susceptibility to some forms of SIDS, which are thought to be caused by failure to arouse from deep sleep to reestablish breathing patterns.

Professor McKenna says that millions of years of cosleeping and night feeding have not developmentally prepared young babies to "sleep through" in a solitary bed, involving, as this does, long periods of deep sleep. Videos taken during the study showed that cosleeping mothers, even in deep sleep, seemed aware of their baby's position and moved when necessary to avoid overlying. At no time in the study did cosleeping mothers impede the breathing of their babies, who actually had higher average oxygen levels than solitary sleepers. Some of the lowest rates of SIDS are found among cultures where cosleeping is predominant.

Western studies indicate that cosleeping does not increase SIDS risk unless cosleeping parents smoke or use alcohol or drugs. Cosleeping parents must ensure that their baby's head does not become covered by bedding, that the baby cannot sink into an overly soft mattress (waterbeds are not recommended), and that the baby does not become entrapped or over-heated.

Fathers, non-breastfeeding mothers, and working parents may particularly appreciate the cozy intimacy that sleeping with a baby brings. Though cosleeping isn't a cure-all for fatigue, many families find it is easier, more pleasurable, and less tiring than our culture's usual sleeping arrangements.

This arrangement, in my experience, allowed me to breastfeed my babies without having to fully awaken. The warmth of my body was just the right temperature for them. We could respond quickly to cries or other needs. The babies could nurse frequently, giving them more antibodies to fight disease.

Dr. McKenna goes on to say, "Human infants need constant attention and contact with other human beings because they are unable to look after themselves. Unlike other mammals, they cannot keep themselves warm, move about, or feed themselves until relatively late in life. It is their extreme neurological immaturity at birth and slow maturation that makes the mother-infant relationship so important."

One of my fondest memories is when we were sleeping with our little ones in a family bed. Once, in the middle of the night, my eighteen-month-old daughter awakened to nurse. She looked up into my face and patted my cheek. "I like you, Mommy, I like you," she said, then closed her eyes and went back to sleep with a sweet smile on her face. Every time I remember that moment, my heart fills with love, joy, and gratitude that this child has come into my life.

Dr. McKenna agrees that this type of interaction is beneficial for both parents and infants. He says, "Studies have shown that separation of the mother and infant has adverse consequences. Anthropological considerations also suggest that separation between the mother and infant should be minimal. Western societies must consider carefully how far and under what circumstances they want to push infants away from the loving and protective cosleeping environment. Infants' nutritional, emotional, and social needs as well as maternal responses to them have evolved in this environment for millennia."

Dr. McKenna has written a particularly insightful article on cosleeping for the website *Neuroanthropology,* which he has graciously allowed me to excerpt below:

Unfortunately, the terms cosleeping, bedsharing and a well-known dangerous form of cosleeping, couch or sofa cosleeping, are mostly used interchangeably by medical authorities, even though these terms need to be kept separate. It is absolutely wrong to say, for example, that "cosleeping is dangerous" when roomsharing is a form of cosleeping and this form of cosleeping (as at least three epidemiological studies show) reduce an infant's chances of dying by one half.

Bedsharing is another form of cosleeping which can be made either safe or unsafe, but it is not intrinsically one nor the other. Couch or sofa cosleeping is, however, intrinsically dangerous as babies can and do all too easily get pushed against the back of the couch by the adult, or flipped face down in the pillows, to suffocate.

Often news stories talk about "another baby dying while cosleeping" but they fail to distinguish between what type of cosleeping was involved and, worse, what specific dangerous factor might have actually been responsible for the baby dying. A specific example is whether the infant was sleeping prone next to their parent, which is an independent risk factor for death regardless of where the infant was sleeping. Such reports inappropriately suggest that all types of cosleeping are the same, dangerous, and all the practices around cosleeping carry the same high risks, and that no cosleeping environment can be made safe.

Nothing can be further from the truth. This is akin to suggesting that because some parents drive drunk with their infants in their cars, unstrapped into car seats, and because some of these babies die in car accidents that nobody can drive with babies in their cars because obviously car transportation for infants is fatal. You see the point.

One of the most important reasons why bedsharing occurs, and the reason why simple declarations against it will not eradicate it, is because sleeping next to one's baby is biologically appropriate, unlike placing infants prone to sleep or putting an infant in a room to sleep by itself. This is particularly so when bedsharing is associated with breast feeding.

When done safely, mother-infant cosleeping saves infants' lives and contributes to infant and maternal health and well being. Merely having an infant sleeping in a room with a committed adult caregiver (cosleeping) reduces the chances of an infant dying from SIDS or from an accident by one half!

Dr. McKenna goes on to cite research conducted in Japan on cosleeping and breastfeeding:

In Japan where cosleeping and breastfeeding (in the absence of maternal smoking) is the cultural norm, rates of the sudden infant death syndrome are the lowest in the world. For breastfeeding mothers, bedsharing makes breastfeeding much easier to manage and practically doubles the amount of breastfeeding sessions while permitting both mothers and infants to spend more time asleep. The increased exposure to mother's antibodies which comes with more frequent nighttime breastfeeding can potentially, per any given infant, reduce infant illness. And because cosleeping in the form of bedsharing makes breastfeeding easier for mothers, it encourages them to breastfeed for a greater number of months, according to Dr. Helen Ball's studies at the University of Durham, therein potentially reducing the mothers' chances of breast cancer.

Furthermore, Dr. McKenna addresses concerns many parents have about bedsharing:

There is no doubt that bedsharing should be avoided in particular circumstances and can be practiced dangerously. While each single bedsharing death is tragic, such deaths are no more indictments about any and all bedsharing than are the three hundred thousand plus deaths or more of babies in cribs an indictment that crib sleeping is deadly and should be eliminated. Just as unsafe cribs and unsafe ways to use cribs can be eliminated so, too, can parents be educated to minimize bedsharing risks.

Cosleeping may not be an option everyone chooses, but I encourage you to read up on it before deciding. It can contribute immensely to implementing the values we hold dear with infant massage. My favorite book on the subject is *The Family Bed* by Tine Thevenin. Of course, Dr. McKenna's book *Sleeping with Your Baby: A Parent's Guide to Cosleeping* is also an invaluable source.

Carrying

Some babies just need a lot of in-arms time, and the vast array of front packs and slings now available make it easier for both parents to respond to a baby's need for closeness. In one study, mothers of newborns were divided into two groups: one group was given plastic infant seats, the other one baby carrier packs. At three months, the babies who had been carried often in the soft carriers (facing the parent) looked more often at their mothers and cried less than those who had spent most of their time in infant seats. At thirteen months, the carried babies were more likely to be securely attached to their parents than the infant seat group.

Carrying an infant in a pack also provides the benefits of stimulating the baby's gastrointestinal system, slowing the heart rate, promoting more effective respiratory functioning, and decreasing congestion. Moreover, the familiar rhythms and rocking of a parent's body going about his or her daily activities are soothing and calming. As Terry Levy and Michael Orlans note in their book *Attachment, Trauma, and Healing,* "Infants who are placed in heart-to-heart proximity with a primary caregiver maintain a mutual heart synchrony."

In addition, carrier packs soothe babies by allowing them to stay warm and to feel as well as listen to their parent's heartbeat. Heartbeat sounds have been shown to increase appetite and thus weight gain, to regulate sleep and respiration, and to reduce crying by 50 percent.

Research published in the journal *Current Biology* shows that infants experience an automatic calming reaction when they are being carried, whether they are mouse pups or human babies. Kumi Kuroda of the RIKEN Brain Science Institute in Saitama, Japan, says, "From humans to mice, mammalian infants become calm and relaxed when they are carried by their mother."

Being held in a parent's arms is the safest place for a baby to be, and parents can have peace of mind knowing their baby is happy, content, and relaxed. The fact that babies are neurobiologically wired to stop crying when carried is a part of the evolutionary biology that helps our species survive.

According to an article in *ScienceDaily,* Kuroda's study "is the first to show that the infant calming response to carrying is a coordinated set of central, motor, and cardiac regulations that is an evolutionarily preserved aspect of mother-infant interactions." It also helps to have a scientific explanation for the frustration many new parents struggle with—a calm and relaxed infant will often begin crying immediately when he or she is put down.

With my newborns, swaddling them created a compact posture and a sense of security that triggered a relaxation response when they were put back down. After I had massaged them every day for a few weeks, using Touch Relaxation (a conditioned response), massage time was another way they relaxed, and their sleep came sooner and was deeper than before.

Kuroda and colleagues determined that the calming response is mediated by the parasympathetic nervous system and a region of the brain called the cerebellum. The researchers found that the calming response was dependent on tactile inputs and proprioception—the ability to sense and understand body movements and keep track of your body's position in space. They also found that the parasympathetic nervous system helped lower the heart rate as part of mediating the coordinated response to being carried. Both human and mouse babies usually calm down and stop moving after they are carried, and mouse pups stop emitting ultra-high-pitched cries.

The idea that the familiar calming dynamic was also playing out in mice occurred to Kuroda one day when she was cleaning the cages of her mouse colony in the laboratory. She says, "When I picked the pups up at the back skin very softly and swiftly as mouse mothers did, they immediately stopped moving and became compact. They appeared relaxed, but not totally floppy, and kept the limbs flexed. This calming response in mice appeared similar to me to soothing by carrying in human babies."

Scientists have known for years that the cerebellum is directly linked to a feedback loop with the vagus nerve, which keeps the heart rate slow and gives you grace under pressure. As adults, we can calm ourselves by practicing mindfulness and meditation, which puts the cerebellum at peace and creates a parasympathetic response of well-being. This appears to be the same response that occurs in infants when they are being carried.

The only time when the cerebellum is allowed to let down its guard and go offline is during REM sleep, when your body is paralyzed to prevent you from acting out your dreams. It makes sense that being picked up and carried would send automatic signals that allow the cerebellum to relax and create healthy vagal tone, which would lower heart rates in infants.

The researchers believe that these findings could have broad implications for parenting and may contribute to preventing child abuse. "This infant response reduces the maternal burden of carrying and is beneficial for both the mother and the infant," explains Kuroda. She goes on to say, "Such proper understanding of infants would reduce frustration of parents and be beneficial, because unsoothable crying is a major risk factor for child abuse.

"A scientific understanding of this infant response will save parents from misreading the restart of crying as the intention of the infant to control the parents, as some parenting theories—such as the 'cry it out' type of strategy—suggest," Kuroda says. "Rather, this phenomenon should be interpreted as a natural consequence of the infant sensorimotor systems." If parents understand that properly, perhaps they will be less frustrated by the crying, writes Kuroda. And that puts those children at lower risk of abuse.

Vocalization

Another element in the dance of bonding is vocalization. From the moment she first responded to sound at around seven months gestation, your infant has been listening to your voice. Her body moves in rhythm with your speech patterns, and the high-pitched tone you use when talking to her is particularly sweet to her ears. During her massage, you might sing a song or tell a story. She will come to associate certain sounds with the massage. Repeat her name and say the word "relax" to gently teach her how to release tension. (We'll cover this more in Chapter 9.)

Infant massage helps enhance the bond begun at birth. A baby learns to enjoy the wonderful comfort and security of loving and being loved. He acquires knowledge about his own body as his parent shows him how to relax a tense arm or leg, or helps him to release painful gas. His parent looks into his eyes, sings, talks soothingly, and gently strokes his skin. Thus each day the dance of bonding begins all over again.

"I feel much closer to my baby and more in tune with her body," says Debbie, mother of three-month-old Kelly. "Knowing that she is growing so fast, it is precious to be able to keep in touch with her little body and experience her growth day by day. I think she feels closer to me also, and there is a real trust developing because of our daily massage. I want to treasure her infancy with all its joys and problems. Massage is a wonderful way for me to do that. The benefits to my baby—physically and emotionally—are extra gifts."

Research from the University of Maryland and Harvard University published in the *Journal of Child Language* suggests that young infants benefit from hearing words repeated by their parents. With this knowledge, parents may make conscious communication choices that could pay off in their babies' toddler years and beyond. "Parents who repeat words more often to their infants have children with better language skills a year and a half later," says study coauthor Rochelle Newman, professor and chair of the University of Maryland's Department of Hearing and Speech Sciences (HESP). "A lot of recent focus has been on simply talking more to your child—but how you talk to your child matters. It isn't just about the number of words."

"Both the child and the parent play a role in the child's later language outcomes, and our study is the first to show that," says HESP professor Nan Bernstein Ratner. While it is clinically proven that parents naturally speak more slowly and in a specialized "singsong" tone to their children, the findings from this study will perhaps encourage parents to be more conscious of repeating words to maximize language development benefits.

A U.S. study shows that the repetitive babbles of babies are primarily motivated by the infants' ability to hear themselves. "Hearing is a critical aspect of infants' motivation to make early sounds," says study author Mary Fagan, an assistant professor of communication science and disorders in the University of Missouri School of Health Professions. "The fact that they attend to and learn from their own behaviors, especially in speech, highlights how infants' own experiences help their language, social and cognitive development," she adds. This research, Fagan says, does not diminish the importance of the speech that babies hear from others.

Odor

New mothers' brains are wired so that the scent of their babies helps them handle the often difficult first few months of motherhood. Research indicates that new moms, given clothes that were worn by infants, detected their babies and had significant changes in their prefrontal cortex—the "seat of sober second thought." The scent of your baby is a natural inducement to help you to cope with the demands of new motherhood. Canadian research found that an infant's smell raises levels of the neurotransmitter dopamine, the "pleasure messenger," in the center of the brain.

Because taste and smell are important to the bonding process, I urge you to use unscented, organic oil when massaging your little one. Your baby will absorb the oil into the skin, and will taste it as he mouths his hands.

Engagement

"Engagement" just means that you are fully present with your baby. Some ideas that can help you be engaged involve talking and singing to your little one.

Talking

Your touch can help your baby learn the words in your language. Research from Purdue University shows that a parent's touch can help babies find words in the continuous stream of speech. "We found that infants treat touches as if they are related to what they hear and thus these touches could have an impact on their word learning," says Amanda Seidl, an associate professor of speech, language, and hearing sciences who studies language acquisition. "We think of touch as conveying affection, but our recent research shows that infants can relate touches to their incoming speech signal. Others have looked at the role of touch with respect to babies forming an attachment and physical development. But until now the impact of touch on language learning has not been explored. Parents may pause before saying an infant's name, but they almost never do so for other words. This research explored whether touches could help infants to find where words begin and end in the continuous stream of speech. They need to find words before they can attach real meaning to their words," Seidl says. "Because names of body parts are often the first words that babies learn and touching is often involved when caregivers talk about body parts, we speculated that touch could act as a cue to word edges."

This information is yet another positive benefit of infant massage. Parents can identify the baby's body parts as they move through the massage. Using the phrase "I love you!" when doing the stroke on the baby's belly is universally stimulating, and often as babies grow older they will say the phrase with Mom or Dad.

Gaze Shifting

Babies learn language best by interacting with people rather than passively through a video or audio recording. But it's unclear which aspects of social interactions make them so important for learning. One study says that an early social behavior called "gaze shifting" is linked to infants' ability to learn sounds of new languages. Gaze shifting, when a baby makes eye contact with a person and then looks at the same object that the other person is looking at, is one of the earliest social skills that babies show.

"We found that the degree to which infants visually tracked the tutors and the toys they held was linked to brain measures of infant learning, showing that social behaviors give helpful information to babies in a complex natural language learning situation," says neuroscientist Patricia Kuhl, the author of the research. "These moments of shared visual attention develop as babies interact with their parents, and they change the baby's brain," adds coauthor Rechele Brooks.

"Our findings show that young babies' social engagement contributes to their own language learning—they're not just passive listeners of language. They're paying attention, and showing parents they're ready to learn when they're looking back and forth. That's when the most learning happens," Brooks says.

"Babies learn best from people. During playtime your child is learning so much from you. Spending time with your child matters. Keeping them engaged—that's what helps them learn language," Brooks concludes. While you are massaging, you can, for example, hold your baby's foot and say, "Foot!" while looking back and forth between baby and her foot. Eventually you'll hear your baby say, "Foot!"

According to another study, the way a newborn gazes may have something to do with how his or her behavior will turn out later on. Researchers from Birkbeck, University of London, say that a newborn's gaze may predict if the baby will grow up into a hyperactive child. Researchers found that babies who tend to focus on an image for a short period of time were more likely to become hyperactive during childhood, compared to babies who hold their gaze on the image for longer periods.

"We were struck that differences between newborns in their visual attention predicted how the children would behave when they were older," says study author Angelica Ronald, according to a *Live Science* report. Researchers also found that children who have shorter focus time tend to exhibit other types of behavioral issues.

According to the study, the differences found in babies may be due to genetics or the kind of environment they have been exposed to while still inside the womb. It was added that a child's ability to focus visually is not just influenced by parental involvement. Even if the ability to pay attention depends on genetic factors, Ronald says, it is still possible for people to learn how to improve their attention span.

Singing

In our infant massage classes, we incorporate parents singing to their babies as soon as the parents feel confident in delivering many of the strokes.

When I was developing our program, I found that singing a slow, repetitive, rhythmic lullaby helped both me and my baby to relax and have fun with the massage. I believe it is an important part of the parent-infant bonding that is the cornerstone of infant massage, and I believe that recent studies, such as the one described below, confirm that assumption. This is a break from traditional Indian baby massage, which is often performed in silence.

A study by researcher Shannon Delecroix investigates how a mother's singing may teach her baby to control his emotions. Delecroix has spent years studying how a mother's music can influence a child's development. She found that "infant-directed singing" does more than create a bond; it helps babies learn focus and self-control. "It also helps babies modulate their arousal level," she says, "so they're not over- or under-aroused; they're kind of 'in the zone.'"

One parent says that music helps her structure her infant's day. "It's a cue to her when we're going to start different activities," she says. "I have certain songs I sing to her when we're going to start different activities; I have certain songs I sing to her in the morning so she knows it's time to wake up, others I sing to her at night when it's time to go to bed."

In another study, researchers used a Jolly Jumper to study the emergence of something called "rhythmic entrainment." Babies are outfitted with motion sensors and then exposed to various types of music and tempos. Delecroix says, "The way the infant responds to a particular musical stimulus tells us a lot about how the human brain is wired."

From the moment I incorporated a rhythmic lullaby into our daily massage, I knew it was important. It structures the massage, because singing this lullaby—the one we use most often is the Bengali lullaby "Ami Tomake Balobhasi Baby" (meaning "I love you, my baby" in the Bengali language)—has a rhythm that goes beautifully with the rhythm of the strokes. These studies confirmed for me that our singing of "Ami Tomake" is spot-on.

According to a study published in the journal *Philosophical Transac-*

tions of the Royal Society, babies have some important lessons to share about bonding and the power of music. The findings show that music has important social effects on infants—as long as the little ones and their parents aren't just listening passively, says Laura Cirelli, the study's lead author and a researcher at McMaster University in Hamilton, Ontario.

"There's this idea that if we just play music in the background, then our kids are going to grow up to be geniuses, and that's really not what research is suggesting," Cirelli says. "If there are benefits of musical activities, it really comes from active engagement in the music." Many families already use music to engage with their kids. The study suggests that "when parents are singing lullabies to infants and rocking them, the babies are actually thinking about them, too," Cirelli says. The same goes for infant massage.

According to Sophie Freeman in an article for the *Daily Mail,* "Researchers found that infants remained relaxed for twice as long when listening to a song—even if it was unfamiliar—as they did when listening to speech." This is interesting news for infant massage, indicating that our use of a rhythmic lullaby will soothe and calm the baby being massaged, even more than talking to the baby.

Professor Isabelle Peretz, from McGill University's Centre for Research on Brain, Language, and Music, says, "Our findings leave little doubt about the efficacy of singing nursery rhymes for maintaining infants' composure for extended periods." She added that singing might reduce feelings of frustration felt by some parents.

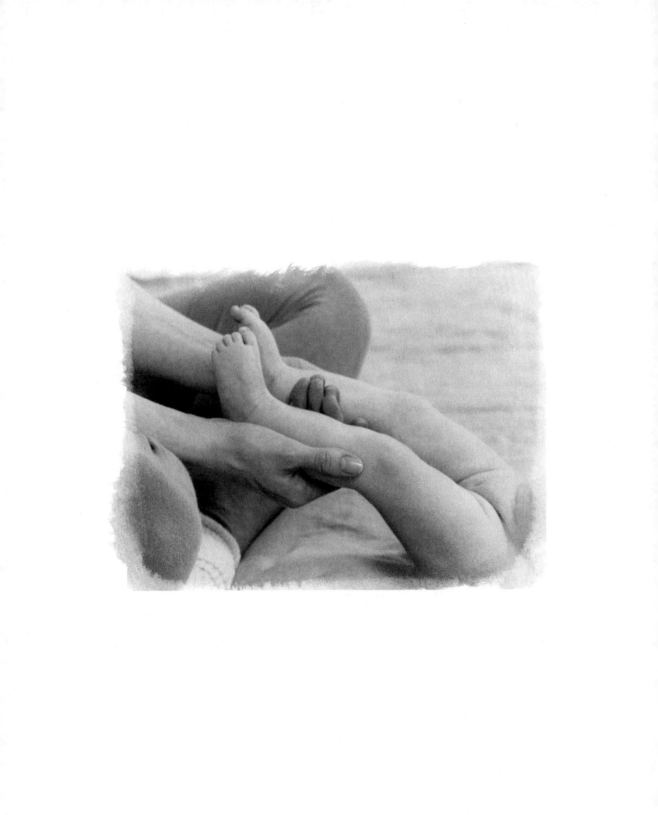

Chapter 7

Attachment and the Benefits of Infant Massage

Keep your life simple,
and serenity will follow.

Like a small country with little
need for supersonic travel,
a simple life has little need for
tension and stress.

Give your children yourself, and
the need for things will be minimal.

—VIMALA MCCLURE,

THE TAO OF MOTHERHOOD

What Is Attachment?

Another word often used in connection with bonding is attachment. While bonding is specific to birth and our connection with the animal kingdom, attachment happens over time and can occur between any two beings. Frank Bolton in his book *When Bonding Fails* describes bonding as a one-directional process that begins in the biological mother during pregnancy and continues through birth and the first days of her baby's life. Conversely, attachment is an interaction between parents and children, biological or not, that develops during the first year they are together and is reinforced throughout life. He describes it as the feeling that the other is "irreplaceable."

Often the terms *bonding* and *attachment* are used interchangeably, because in humans the bonding period is so loosely defined as to merge into the attachment process. According to researcher John Kennell, "An attachment can be defined as a unique emotional relationship between two individuals which is specific and endures through time." That definition could also apply to the word *bonding*. In this book, I am using these terms interchangeably as well, as we are not conforming here to strict research or medically oriented language. Rather, we use these concepts in our everyday speech to imply the love that develops between parent and child, whether the child is a birth parent's newborn or an adopted baby or toddler. Bonding and attachment, as we use the terms, are the whole continuum of closeness that happens over time and that can be augmented by the practice of infant massage.

Kennell and his colleague Marshall Klaus cited cuddling, kissing, and prolonged gazing as indicators of a developing bond. Dramatic evidence in their studies and others correlates the lack of early bonding and attachment with later abuse, neglect, and failure to thrive. Mothers who are separated from their babies during the newborn period are often more hesitant to learn and unskilled in basic mothering tasks. Even very short separations sometimes adversely affect the relationship between mothers and infants.

Experts in many fields are becoming increasingly alarmed at what has been termed the "bonding crisis" in Western countries. Long before the outbreak of violence among children in the United States, Dr. Ken Magid, psychologist and author of *High Risk: Children Without a Conscience,* pointed to what he called a "profound demographic revolution" that is changing the course of history. "Working mothers—and the possibility that their children are suffering bonding breaks—are simply not being given enough attention," he says. In 1988, in a chilling foretelling of events to come, he cited the stresses of two-income families, single parents struggling to survive, an achievement-addicted society, poorly run and understaffed day care facilities, little or no parental leave in the job market, poorly handled adoptions, and inadequate child custody arrangements following divorce as risk factors for our newest generations of infants.

Secure Attachment

Research shows that simply touching or caressing a newborn is critical to the infant's sense of security. Infant massage, therefore, becomes an incredibly important art for parents to learn. Usually it is the mother who is the central focus of studies like these, probably because the mother is often the main caregiver, especially in infancy. But a study at the University of Iowa concludes that "being attached to Dad is just as helpful as being close to Mom." A similar study in 2012 from Imperial College London found that fathers were especially important in helping the infant avoid behavioral problems later in life. If the father is remote or distracted, the child is more likely to be aggressive.

What these studies show is the importance of those first few months of life, when a tiny baby is set on a trajectory that will partly determine success at something as simple—and critical—as getting along with others.

In another article about this research, Lauren Jimeson says, "These studies prove that those first few months of your child's life, when life can be overwhelming and it can be a major adjustment for everyone, are the most critical. It's important that both parents take the time that they need to really focus on being a parent and showing that immense love to your child. Hold them, cuddle them, rock them to sleep, do whatever you can that makes life happy for you and your baby. It's this love that will help shape your child's life forever."

In Dimitri Ehrlich's *The Daddy Diaries,* a blog he writes for the *Huffington Post,* Ehrlich offers an interesting and humorous look at the phenomenon, which he has graciously allowed me to share with you:

Before you have a baby, everyone warns you to kiss sleep goodbye. "Good luck," they say, with a smile full of schadenfreude. (I wonder why German is the only language with a word that means being happy when other people suffer.) They wish you luck the way someone who has just assembled a piece of IKEA furniture says good luck. Like, "I suffered beyond imagination to make something so wobbly I have to lean it against the wall, but at least now I can sit back and laugh while you discover this Riktig Ogla is never going to fit into that Grundtal Norrviken. But go ahead. Good luck."

After all the warnings, I was duly scared about the sleep thing. And it's true. I have not slept more than a few hours in a row for months. But what nobody tells you is how much joy you feel.

I just got up to pick up the baby and I realized that all my fears of being exhausted never materialized. Because when you lean into his crib and he sees you, he erupts into a smile like you just told him he won the $80 million Powerball lottery. That happens multiple times a day. His joy is so overwhelming and infectious that it's impossible to feel tired or beleaguered. It's like a tractor beam of sunlight hitting you in the face. It's like drinking fresh squeezed orange juice. It's like the opening chords of Stevie Wonder's "Sir Duke." It's like the first day of spring after a long cold winter. And it never gets tired.

There is a Buddhist prayer we recite every day, which says, "Regardless of whether conditions seem favorable or unfavorable, inspire me to make a habit of happiness." The other key teaching of Buddha is to love without being attached. And if you thought avoiding attachment was hard with romantic love, it's well nigh impossible with a baby.

Non-attachment doesn't mean being a robot and having no human emotions. It means discerning between the warm, open-hearted side of pure love, and the sticky ego-influenced desire to control another person, a situation, or life in general. That sticky aspect is the glue that binds us to suffering. It causes us to cling and destroys our happiness. So the real challenge of parenthood is to experience these incredible surges of joy without allowing a habit of clinging to immediately follow in equal measure. . . . For that, the Buddha prescribed medicine—meditations of various kinds. But meditation works slowly and this tsunami of love and attachment doesn't knock gently at the front door. It tears the house down.

As they learn about infant massage, parents often make a choice to bond with their babies in whatever way they can. I've had many parents in my classes (instructors, too) who had difficult relationships with their parents in childhood. They read this book, come to classes and seminars, and become acutely aware of their own bonding or lack of it—and they are amazed and grateful for the opportunity to turn things around.

Building a Secure Attachment Bond with Your Baby

The secure attachment bond is the nonverbal emotional relationship between an infant and parent, defined by emotional responses to the baby's cues, as expressed through movements, gestures, and sounds. The success of this wordless relationship enables a baby to feel secure enough to develop fully, and affects how he or she will interact, communicate, and form relationships throughout life. By understanding how you can better participate in this emotional interaction, you can ensure that your child has the best possible foundation for life.

The attachment bond is the unique emotional relationship between your baby and you as his or her parent. This interactive emotional exchange draws the two of you together, ensuring that your infant will feel safe and be calm enough to allow optimal development of her nervous system. The attachment bond is a key factor in the way your infant's brain organizes itself and influences your child's social, emotional, intellectual, and physical development.

Skin-to-skin contact lets babies know that they're safe and protected, building trust between parent and infant. Through the physical contact with adults, strong attachments can be created, thus providing a stable foundation for future relationships. Oxytocin, known as the "bonding hormone," is released during times of close physical contact such as breastfeeding and infant massage.

The quality of the attachment bond varies. A secure bond provides your baby with an optimal foundation for life: eagerness to learn, healthy self-awareness, trust, and consideration for others. An insecure or anxious attachment bond, one that fails to meet your infant's need for safety and understanding, can lead to confusion about her own identity and difficulties in learning and relating to others in later life.

Children need to be able to engage in a nonverbal emotional exchange with their parents in a way that communicates their needs and makes them feel understood, secure, and balanced. Children who feel emotionally disconnected from their parents are likely to feel confused, misunderstood, and insecure.

While it's easiest to form a secure attachment bond when your child is still an infant and reliant upon nonverbal means of communicating, you can begin to make your child feel understood and secure at any age. Children's brains continue maturing well into adulthood. Moreover, because the brain continues to change throughout life, it's never too late to start engaging in a nonverbal emotional exchange with your child.

The attachment process is both interactive and dynamic. You and your baby exchange nonverbal emotional cues that make your baby feel understood and safe. Even in the first days of life, your baby picks up on your emotional cues—your tone of voice, your gestures, and your emotions—and sends you signals by crying, cooing, mimicking facial expressions, and eventually smiling, laughing, pointing, and even screeching and yelling. In return, you watch your baby, listen to her cries and sounds, and respond to her cues at the same time as you tend to her needs for food, warmth, and affection. Secure attachment grows out of the success of this nonverbal communication process between you and your baby.

A secure attachment bond teaches your baby to trust you, to communicate her feelings to you, and eventually to trust others as well. As you and your baby connect with each other, your baby learns how to have a healthy sense of self and how to be in a loving, empathic relationship.

Secure attachment causes the parts of your baby's brain responsible for social and emotional development, communication, and relationships to grow and develop in the best way possible. This relationship becomes the foundation of your child's ability to connect with others in a healthy way. Qualities that you may take for granted in adult relationships—such as empathy, understanding, love, and the ability to be responsive to others—are first learned in infancy.

When babies develop a secure attachment bond, they are better able to:

- Develop fulfilling intimate relationships
- Maintain emotional balance
- Feel confident and good about themselves
- Enjoy being with others
- Rebound from disappointment and loss
- Share their feelings and seek support

Nature has programmed parents as well as their infants to have a "falling in love" experience through attachment. The joy you experience as you connect with your infant goes a long way to relieve fatigue from lack of sleep and the stress of learning how to care for your baby. The bonding process releases endorphins in your body that motivate you, give you energy, and make you feel happy. Creating a secure attachment with your infant may take a little effort, but the rewards are huge for both of you.

Delayed Attachment

Given the appropriate tools and encouragement, a parent and baby can certainly compensate if their bonding has been postponed by separation.

If you were not able to establish intimate, affectionate bonds with your baby early on, don't despair. The beauty of the human species is that we have a marvelous ability to overcome setbacks and learn new patterns. If you are aware of the importance of these bonds, you can find ways to consciously assist nature.

An infant who avoids eye contact, who is stiff and doesn't mold to your body, may need some extra attention and help to begin to trust and form the attachments he needs for healthy development. A daily massage can begin to re-create the elements of bonding that help you get in sync with each other. You may have to start with very little—perhaps only five minutes—and gradually increase as he begins to accept both your stroking and your eye contact. Spending a little extra time carrying him, sleeping with him, taking baths with him, and playing with him when he is active and alert can also help. Whatever activities involve touching, talking, eye contact, and affection are the activities you can focus on. But go slowly. Some parents, in their anxiety at having missed the so-called early bonding window, overcompensate by overstimulating and stressing their baby with too much, too fast. Allow the baby to lead; give your attention, affection, eye contact, cuddling, and carrying in ways he can accept.

Some parents find this re-creation of bonding difficult because of an overload of stress or depression, often caused by separation from their infant. If you feel stressed or depressed, get help now. Counseling can help a great deal; giving voice to pain is an essential means to healing. A counselor or psychotherapist can also help you find ways to deal with stress that you may not have thought about. These days, there are many therapists who specialize in postpartum depression.

In later chapters, we will discuss adoption, fostering, prematurity, and other special situations. Each of these will require a different approach to massage, but none rule it out as part of your parenting routines.

Who Should Massage Your Baby?

Though some neonatal intensive care units (NICUs) have therapists and/or nurses massage the babies, and the massage therapists' organization offers instruction for certified massage therapists in how to massage a baby, it has been important to me, from the very beginning of my teaching, that only parents should massage their infants. In NICUs with fragile premature infants, only parents should be shown by Certified Infant Massage Instructors from IAIM how to use gentle holding methods as a precursor for massage at home. (More about this in Chapter 16.) Our instructors use lifelike dolls to demonstrate strokes for parents in their classes and in coaching parents in the NICU.

Infant massage provides the perfect environment for bonding and secure attachment between parent and infant. It has important physical benefits, too, but they have never been the main consideration. The emotional/psychological bond that continues between parent and baby is the most important reason for infant massage.

Getting to Know Each Other

Regular massage provides a time for a parent to become intimately acquainted with the baby's body language, her rhythms of communication, her thresholds for stimulation, and how her body looks and feels when tense or at ease.

Bonding research also points out that parents feel closer to their infants if they can evoke a positive response from a specific series of actions. Massage, which combines intimacy, communication, play, and caregiving, can greatly enhance a parent's feeling of competence. Setting aside a time for touching and nurturing through massage, a parent sends her baby a very special message that says, "I love you, and I want to communicate with you and you alone." From all my work, I can say that most

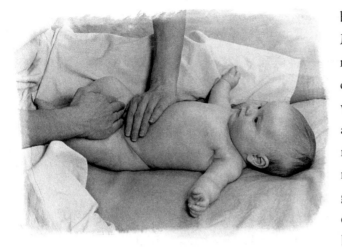

babies do indeed get the message! My own children, grown adults now, continue to benefit from the daily massage routines we had when they were babies. They are affectionate, compassionate, well-rounded human beings. Our closeness has remained throughout their growing years, even the teens and early twenties, when they had to break away to create their own identities and their own paths in life. Though we have had our share of communication breakdowns, we always come back to each other with love—mending, reattaching, and becoming closer and more understanding of one another. Our commitment to our family bond is unbreakable, and I can say unequivocally that I attribute this closeness, our commitment to each other, to our early experiences in building strong attachments through loving, responsive massage.

The Benefits of Infant Massage

The benefits of massaging your baby are many: for your baby, for you as parents, for your family, and for society at large. I have always thought of them as in those categories.

Benefits for Baby
Interaction
Massaging your baby promotes bonding; it contains every element of the bonding process. Infant massage promotes a secure attachment with your child over time. It promotes verbal and nonverbal communication between the two of you. Your baby receives undivided attention from you; he

feels respected and loved. It is one of the only times that all of his senses are nourished.

Stimulation

Infant massage aids in the development of your baby's circulatory, respiratory, and gastrointestinal systems. It aids in sensory integration, helping your baby learn how her body feels and what its limits are. Massaging your baby helps make connections between neurons in the brain, which helps develop her nervous system. It also aids the generation of muscular development and tone, and contributes to her mind/body awareness.

Relaxation

Regular infant massage improves sleep, increases flexibility, and regulates behavioral states. It reduces stress, levels of stress hormones, and hypersensitivity. Massaging your baby creates higher levels of anti-stress hormones and promotes an improved ability to self-calm. It teaches your infant to relax in the face of stress.

Relief

Infant massage helps with gas and colic, constipation and elimination, muscular tension, and teething discomfort. It also helps with growing pains, organizes the nervous system, relieves physical and psychological tension, and softens skin. It helps release physical and emotional tension, balances oxygen levels, and provides a sense of security.

Benefits for Parents

Massaging your baby releases bonding and relaxing hormones into your system. It helps you learn a type of mindfulness ("be here now") as you spend quality time with your infant. It can aid in lactation, self-esteem, and confidence in your parenting. The bonding and secure attachment help you be a better parent. It is a wonderful way for fathers to be intimately involved with the care of their babies, and helps both parents understand their baby's "language."

Benefits for the Family

Infant massage encourages the involvement of siblings and extended family in baby care. It promotes a relaxed environment in the home, communication, and respect.

Benefits for Society

Imagine a world where people are trained to be good parents; where newborns, older babies, toddlers, and children are routinely given healthy, loving massages every day; where the entire culture values positive, nurturing touch, respect, and empathy. There would be reduced infant health care costs, less child abuse, fewer behavioral problems in children, and less violence. When I founded the International Association of Infant Massage, this is what I imagined: changing the world, one baby at a time.

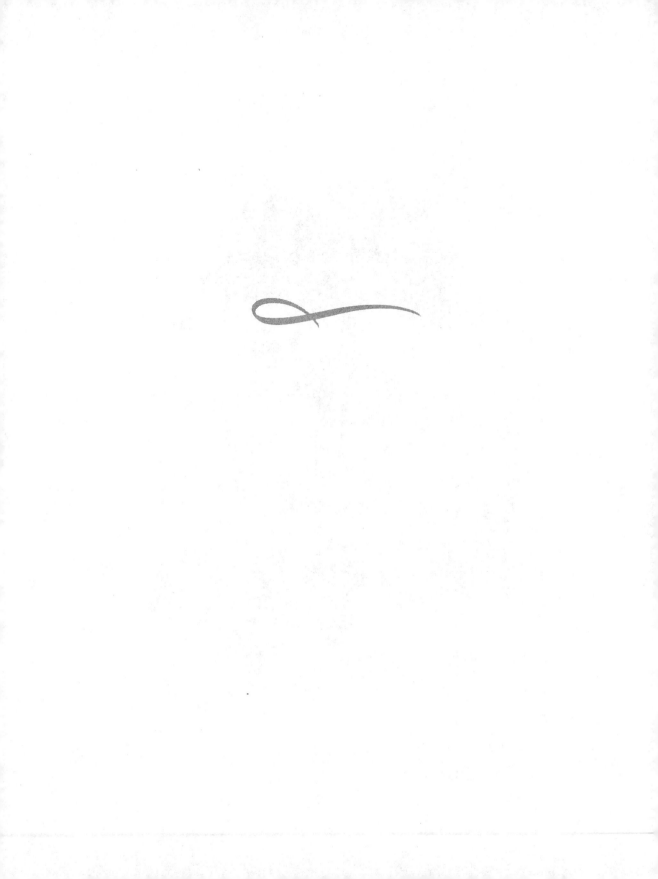

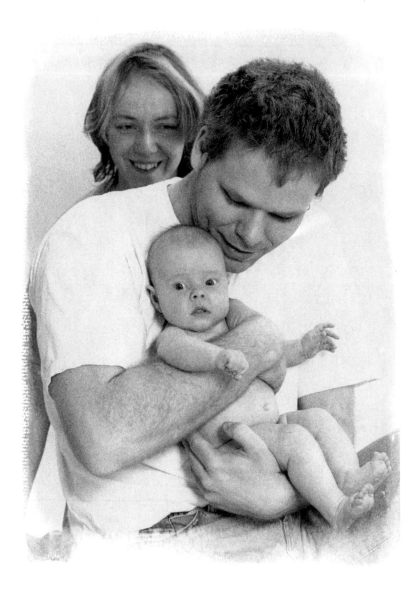

Chapter 8

Especially for Fathers

Our little bud of Paradise
Is wakeful, Father. I suppose
His clever brain already knows
That if he bubbles long enough
His head will lean against the rough
Attraction of your overcoat.

—NORMAN GALE, "HOME FROM BUSINESS"

Dad, Get Involved Right from the Start

Fathers today take an increasingly active interest in the care and nurturing of their infants. However, men often feel dissatisfied with their ability to form this meaningful relationship. Fifty years ago, dads were relegated to the waiting room as the birth of their child took place behind closed doors. Fast-forward to the present, and those doors have been thrown wide open. In many instances, however, fathers are still part of the background, playing supportive but limited roles in the upbringing of their babies. Creating a bond should begin at birth, and research has shown that massage can serve as one of the building blocks for father-child bonds.

Research has found that instruction in infant massage for new dads may substantially influence the quality of their relationship. In one study, fathers who massaged their babies were found to be more demonstrative, warmer, and accepting with their babies. In another instance, the fathers' stress and their participation in an infant massage class were studied. It was found that the classes appreciably decreased the fathers' stress levels; 92 percent had a positive experience. Another study showed that dads acknowledged that infant massage is an extraordinary tool for bonding and a way to become more comfortable with their infants. Still another piece of research on an infant massage class for fathers showed that they had expanded feelings of competency, acceptance of their roles, attachment, support from their partners, and reduced feelings of isolation and depression. According to an article in the *Journal of Perinatal Education*, "Supporting Fathering Through Infant Massage," "infant massage classes appear to offer fathers the positive experience of meeting other fathers and enjoying the opportunity to share their fathering experiences."

In spite of an eagerness to participate in the baby's care right from the beginning, a new father may encounter logistical problems. His time may be limited to evenings and weekends. He may be tired after work. He may have to face the added stress of coping with basic household maintenance and increased financial pressure. Dad may be hard-pressed to find time for himself and may seem withdrawn at times when mother and baby want and need just the opposite response. Of course, Mom is coping with the same problems, compounded by the sometimes overwhelming responsibility of caring for the baby around the clock. Add fatigue from the birth, breastfeeding issues, and raging hormones, and she can be exhausted and seriously in need of some "me time."

Tiffany Field, from the Touch Research Institute in Miami, conducted a study in 2000 that found fathers who massaged their infants were "more expressive and showed more enjoyment and more warmth during floor-play interactions with their infants." Moreover, fathers who participated in massage experienced increased self-esteem as a parent. Field noted that while the dads reaped benefits, their babies also realized some advantages— they tended to greet the fathers with more direct eye contact, and they smiled and vocalized more.

Another study reported in the *Journal of Perinatal Education* yielded similar results after observing two groups of twelve infant-father dyads for four weeks. Fathers in the experimental group massaged their babies, while dads in the control group did not. After massaging their infants, the fathers demonstrated a decrease in their stress scores. The authors conclude that infant massage is a "viable option for teaching fathers caregiving sensitivity." Additionally, the results suggest that fathers who massage their infants experience "increased feelings of competence, role acceptance, spousal support, attachment and health by decreasing feelings of isolation and depression."

In 2013, Mary Kay Keller, a Certified Infant Massage Instructor with IAIM and an author, educator, researcher, and relationship coach, published her dissertation, in which she investigated the benefits fathers perceived as having received from massaging their infants. In addition to increased sensitivity and competency, the dads reported greater awareness that they were contributing to the child's well-being. They were motivated to spend time massaging their infant for two reasons: to give Mom a break and to help decrease stress in the baby. They also valued the opportunity to enjoy their baby and the ultimate bond they were creating. When a bond is forged early on, the chances for a strong, healthy relationship later in life are increased. As men become more actively involved in their children's lives, it is worthwhile to explore the benefits massage can provide for both baby and dad. Keller has also given TED Talks about her findings, which you can view online.

In the first weeks after birth, a mother may be tired at the end of the day, and the baby may be fussy. Far from fitting some people's notion of a stay-at-home mom luxuriating in the playful company of her baby and soap operas on television, the new mother has task after task to perform throughout the day, with no breaks and little contact with other adults. Many tasks are repetitive—cleaning, washing, diapering, feeding, comforting, grocery shopping—and there's not the validation of a paycheck or a pat on the back from a supervisor. So when Dad gets home from his job, most moms aren't necessarily cheery. One father, whose wife died, says he thought he had been very involved with his children before, but "I didn't know how removed I was until I had to do all the thousands and thousands of things it takes to raise a child."

Don't Wait for an Invitation

Dads, don't wait for an invitation to get involved with the care of your baby. At the hospital, birthing center, or home, during the first few days, don't let well-meaning aunts or grandmothers push you out of the way. Ask the nurse or midwife or grandmother how to change, burp, and bathe the baby, and how to take the baby's temperature. If you and your partner have agreed, learn how to feed the baby. (Even breastfed babies can occasionally accept breast milk from a bottle.) If your partner complains about the way you do things, don't be defensive. Ask her to show you how she does it, and thank her. As one dad says, "After a while, she'll get tired of being the 'baby boss' and will relinquish more and more control to you." Studies have shown that a father's sensitive caregiving predicts secure attachment and that a warm, gratifying marital relationship supports fathers' involvement with their babies.

Both parents can be hard-pressed to find time for themselves and their relationship in addition to being good parents. A father may seem withdrawn at times when the mother and baby want and need just the opposite response. This usually means, at least in the beginning, sleep deprivation for both parents.

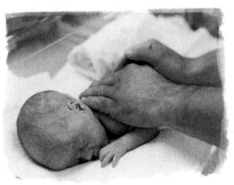

These stressors present fathers with a high barrier in learning to nurture their children with soft and gentle care. So does their lack of learned "maternal" behavior: because most men have not grown to manhood learning the same behaviors toward babies that most women do, they may need special help and encouragement in the beginning.

But fathers can walk, rock, sing to, dance with, read to, and massage their babies as well as feed, change, and bathe them. Many people don't realize that fathers, too, have "parenting hormones" that are activated by close contact with their infants.

Psychologist Tom Daly comments, "In the process of giving the massage, fathers get to know their children in an extraordinary way. They connect with a deep part of the child and with a deep part of themselves—their nurturing side. Boys, by and large, are conditioned to suppress this part by the age of nine, but working with infants in this way opens up that old place. Dads find they are great nurturers when given a safe situation in which their manhood is not compromised."

When fathers give their children extra attention, he notes, the children have more self-confidence and exhibit more creativity. "Men and manhood are changing," Daly says. "Let us continue to get fathers more seriously involved in child rearing. Infant massage is a golden opportunity to assist in this transformation. The world is a better place every time an infant is massaged, and men need to be part of this."

Nurturant Men, Successful Women: You Can Help

Children benefit immensely from affectionate interaction with both parents. "A warm, affectionate father-son relationship can strengthen a boy's masculine development," says Dr. Michael Lamb, author of *The Role of the Father in Child Development*. "A nurturant father is a more available model than a non-nurturant father. The nurturant father's behavior is more often associated with affection and praise and it acquires more reward value. Thus a boy with a nurturant father has more incentive to imitate his father than a boy with a non-nurturant father."

Girls, too, need wholesome bonds with their fathers. The Mills Longitudinal Study indicates that the women who were most healthy and well-adjusted as adults grew up in homes with two loving, involved parents. The most successful women had fathers who valued femininity and encouraged competency, who were both warm and affectionate with their daughters and supportive of their efforts toward independence.

Massage is a quality experience for parents and infants, from which both benefit immensely. The baby learns that Daddy can touch him gently and lovingly, that Daddy, too, is someone he can count on to help meet his physical and emotional needs. A father who realizes these qualities in himself as a result of the massage experience is certain to have his confidence as a parent substantially boosted.

Fathers who massage their babies regularly throughout infancy later recall that massage time with fondness. "I'll never forget how my son would wiggle and smile when he heard the oil swishing in my hands," says Ron, father of seven-month-old Jason. "It's going to be fun to tell him about it when he gets older and to remind him of it when he has his own kids. Heck, maybe someday I'll massage his baby, too!"

Dear Dad

As a new father, you may have to use some creativity to structure your time to allow for the twenty to thirty minutes you will need to massage your baby. The best time is usually the morning of a day off, when you can relax unhurriedly. After learning the basic techniques from your wife, this book, or a class, you should be alone with your baby for the massage. It is better not to have both parents massaging the baby at once, as this can give your infant mixed signals and make him uncomfortable.

In the beginning, proceed very gently, massaging only the legs or back. You may have a sense of being too strong or too inexpert to massage your baby, your hands too big or rough. Nearly everyone is a little clumsy and nervous in the beginning. Start by gently placing your hands over your baby's back or torso and feeling relaxation and love flow through your hands to your baby. You need not even move your hands in the beginning; just feel the connection between the two of you, and concentrate on relaxing your body and letting your love go to him. When that feels more comfortable, you can begin a simple stroking, stopping now and then to just hold and relax. Remember to make all your movements very smooth and slow, almost like slow motion. Talk or sing softly, make eye contact when baby is ready, and in general follow the baby's rhythms of communication. As time goes on and your baby becomes more familiar with your touch, you may want to spend more time and move on to other parts of the body, developing your own special massage techniques. For more ideas and helpful hints, please read on, for this book is meant for you as well.

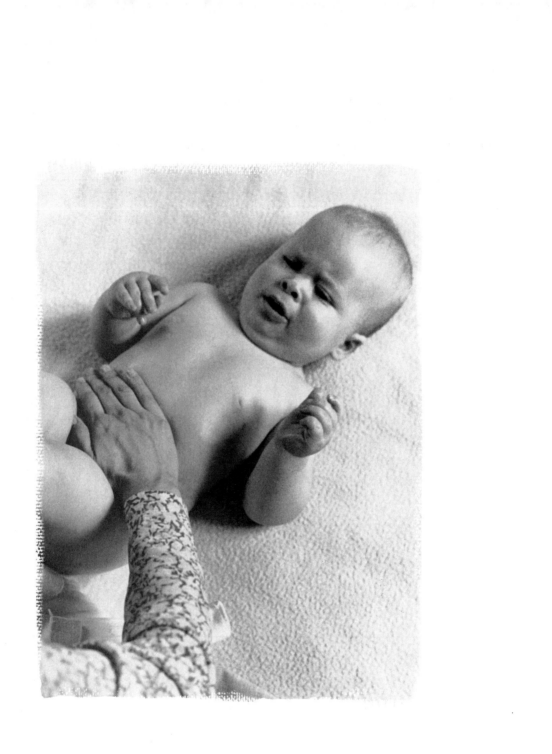

Chapter 9

Helping Baby (and You) Learn to Relax

There was a child went forth every day,
And the first object he look'd upon,
that object he became.

—WALT WHITMAN, FROM *LEAVES OF GRASS*

Visualize a Relaxed Baby, a Relaxed Parent

Close your eyes for a moment and picture your baby. What do you see? Is she awake or sleeping? Crying? Active or placid? Tense or relaxed? Chubby or thin? How does your mental image of her compare with the way she really is right now?

Often we unconsciously form images of ourselves and others, including our children, that are based upon limited experience. For instance, my second baby was ill and hospitalized just after she was born. She came home with a clean bill of health, but for a long time I subconsciously pictured her as fragile and weak. Even when I realized that I still carried my early fears and projected them onto her, it was difficult to change that image. It had become a habitual way of thinking. These habits can directly affect those we think about, especially our children, who depend upon us for a clear reflection of themselves.

As parents' thinking is translated into words and actions, a baby adopts them as her own. Positive visualizations and affirmations can help free us from limiting concepts and give our infants feedback to develop to their full potential. The daily massage is a perfect opportunity to practice positive imagery and verbal feedback. As you massage your baby, picture her relaxing, opening, and letting go of tension. Visualize her happy and healthy. Try to picture her internal organs as you massage: see her heart beating, her lungs healthy, her intestinal system functioning smoothly; imagine the blood as it moves through her veins and arteries, and see your massage facilitating the blood flow to her arms and legs. Praise her relaxation, her beautiful smile, the softness of her skin. Here are a few examples of statements that help babies adopt positive attitudes about themselves:

"How nice and soft your tummy is!"

"I can feel the gas bubbles moving. Can you help push them out?"

"You are learning to relax your legs. That's wonderful!"

"Ah, so relaxed, so loose. You feel so happy now."

"Sarah helps Mommy massage. Such a big girl!"

Are You Relaxed?

The first few months of your baby's life are happy and exciting, but they can also be stressful. Right now, take an inventory of your body. Which areas are tense? Are you breathing deeply and fully? Perhaps you are holding your baby, nursing, or walking about as you read. Is your baby fussy? When he cries, what happens to your body? Do you tense up, hold your breath, or breathe shallowly? If your baby is sleeping, are you anxious or restive, partially alert for his cries?

The miraculous changes you have undergone during pregnancy and delivery, the demands of caring for a new baby, and the lack of sleep and quiet time all add up to tension and anxiety, which can become habitual in the early weeks and months of parenthood. Your baby's daily massage offers a time to relax and unwind. In fact, a relaxed state of mind is essential.

Fussy Time of Day?

At one time or another, every mother has felt tense and nervous, and in spite of her best efforts the baby begins to fuss and cry. Babies are wonderfully sensitive little beings who pick up every nuance of your communication. If you say "relax" with a furrowed brow, the baby will get both messages, but the furrowed brow is much more meaningful to him than your words.

Perhaps your baby has a fussy period during the day or evening. An hour or so before it usually begins, massage him to provide him with an outlet for built-up tension. A simple fifteen-minute massage will be a welcome respite from the cycle of fussy baby, tense mother.

In my son's early infancy, I discovered that massaging him, followed by taking a warm bath together, helped both of us avoid late afternoon or early evening irritability. In the summertime, a massage in the warm morning sun and a splash in the wading pool (made warm by adding hot water from the kitchen) gave me time for quiet, observant meditation and afforded my baby a wonderful sensory experience.

Controlled Belly Breathing

In the many years of my own practice and teaching, I developed a technique I call Controlled Belly Breathing, which I do upon waking and again as I go to sleep at night. This practice can be very beneficial in relaxing and releasing tension, either to get ready for your day or to prepare for a restful night's sleep. It can be quite helpful when your baby is ill and you are not able to get the sleep you need, or as a way to stay flowing with the everyday chaos that a family naturally brings with it.

I suggest you give this a try for at least a month, to see if it makes a difference in your life. Controlled Belly Breathing is easy to do and easy to incorporate into your routine, and if someday you wish to make a practice of daily meditation, mindfulness, or prayer, this is wonderful preparation.

And you can use it at virtually any time—in the car, on a bus, while cooking, before a meeting. It is especially helpful in preparation for potentially stressful events such as dental work or surgery, and before something or someone comes at you with confrontative energy. (Many therapists recommend similar practices for people who have anxiety disorders or panic attacks.) You can use it when your child's behavior has you at the end of your rope and you are so tired and upset you don't know what to do. You can also use it just before the massage routine, as a way of calming yourself and focusing on your love for your baby. Here's how it works:

1. Sit anywhere you like, with your back relatively straight. Your eyes can be open or closed. Breathe out, releasing all of the air in your lungs.
2. Now slowly breathe in, through your nose, to a count of four ("One and two and three and four").
3. Slowly release the air from your lungs at the same pace ("One and two and three and four").
4. Repeat the entire in-out cycle for three minutes, timing yourself with a clock. Try to relax your body more and more as you breathe.

You will notice a slight pause at the end of each cycle, in and out. Let it be there. Don't force the technique, but imagine that the air is "breathing you." Breathe from the very bottom of your belly, allowing your belly to expand as the air comes in and contract as it goes out. During this time, you may say to yourself "relax," or any other word that comes to mind that helps you relax your body and release your mind of worries, cares, and lists. Notice any part of your body that is tense, and consciously relax that area. Some people like to say "slow down," others "let go," but you can simply use the counting as described above if you like.

Touch Relaxation

One of the best things a parent can do for her child is to teach him to help himself. The ability to completely relax is a skill we all could use, and the earlier your child learns it, the more naturally it will come when he needs it. One of the most profound benefits of daily massage that I have seen in my children is the relaxed way they carry themselves, the looseness of their bodies. They became ideal "demonstration models" for me in my classes because of the way they relaxed, even as active toddlers. Even now, as adults, they carry themselves in a relaxed and confident way, I believe because they were massaged every day—sometimes twice a day—when they were babies. Children who have been taught Touch Relaxation techniques in infancy continue to respond as they get older.

Touch Relaxation techniques—used between massage strokes, between sets of strokes, and after finishing the massage—are simple and easy to do. They fit in beautifully with the massage routine, but can also be done at other times. If you attended childbirth preparation classes, you may remember how you consciously rehearsed relaxing each part of your body. You will be using a similar principle with your baby, calling her attention to an area, showing her how to relax it, then giving her positive feedback as she learns.

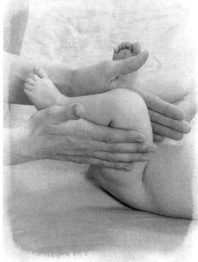

For example, let's say you are beginning to massage the baby's leg, and it appears stiff and tense. Take the leg gently in your hands, encompassing it and molding your hand to the baby's leg. Feel a heavy relaxation in your hand as it conforms to your baby's skin. Now, gently bounce the leg, repeating in a soft voice, "Relax," stressing and elongating the vowel sounds ("Reee-laaaaax"). Use the same tone each time you say this. As soon as you feel any relaxation in the muscles, give the baby some feedback, saying, "Wonderful! You relaxed your leg," and offer a smile and a kiss. The same thing can be done with other parts of the body. To loosen up the tense area, use very gentle rolling, bouncing, and encompassing motions, giving positive feedback when you get a favorable response. Not only will this help the baby focus her attention on her own body so that later she knows how to relax herself, it will also help her to associate your touch with the positive benefits of relaxation.

Resting Hands

Sometimes at the beginning, especially with a medically fragile, premature, or colicky baby, and at different times during the massage, it is helpful to use a simple holding technique. Warming your hands, you simply place them either on or around (cupping) the baby's body. Let your hands go very heavy and warm. Intentionally relax your own body and slow down your breathing. Imagine healing and relaxation flowing through your hands to your baby. See if you can warm up your hands by just using the power of your mind and deeply relaxing your body.

I believe every massage should begin this way, to help both parent and baby slow down and relax into the gentle love of conscious, healthy touch.

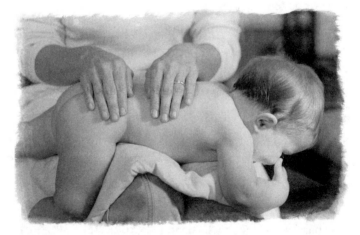

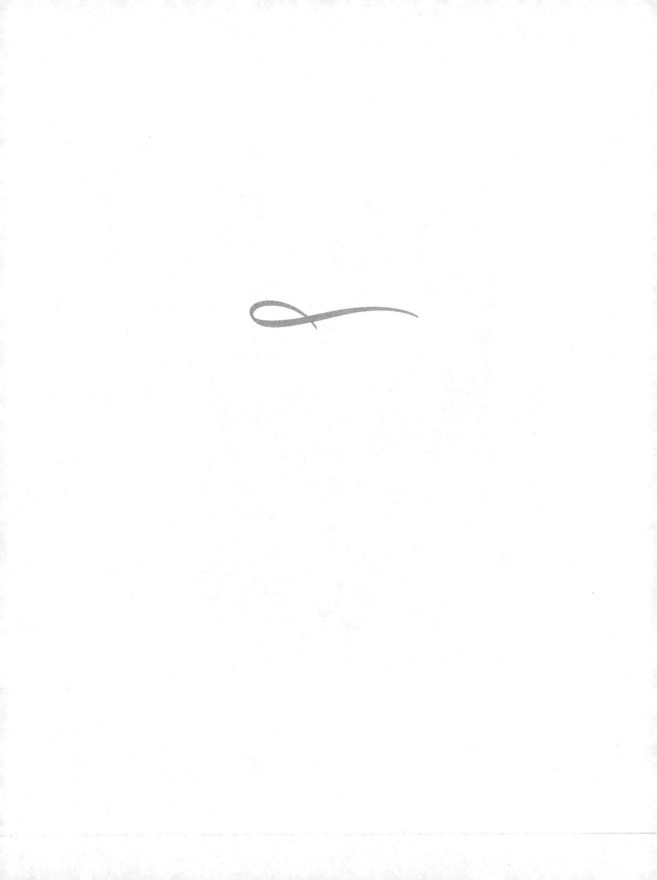

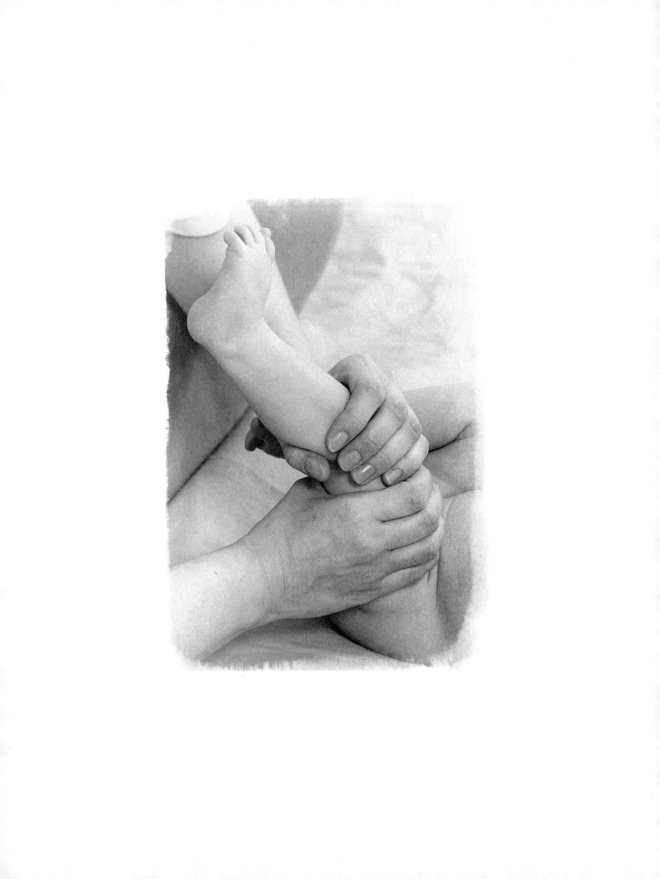

Chapter 10

Your Baby's Brain

*The wise remain aware of the
spirituality of life.*

*Every mother has felt the
stillness and the stir of Eternal
Consciousness in her womb.
Remember that.*

*Bring that mysterious, silent moment
into the clamoring present.*

—VIMALA MCCLURE,

THE TAO OF MOTHERHOOD

Infant Brain Development

Most parents have the best of intentions, but it can be difficult to know which way to step when it comes to doing the very best we can for our children. Science is making it a little easier, with technology that makes it possible to study the developing brain. Parenting, like all things, has gone through its phases, but modern beliefs and practices might be hindering healthy brain and emotional development in children. Parent-infant interactions help foster the neurodevelopment of brain regions producing oxytocin, thus enhancing children's future social and emotional development.

The development of an unborn baby's brain is fascinating, and it helps us understand the amazing benefits of massaging your baby. Knowing how your infant's brain is handling all of the new things surrounding him enables you to approach him with both knowledge and compassion. Drs. Eileen and Tom Paris contend that part of creating a healthy relationship with our children is owning our feelings and expressing them as our own. They say, "For example, telling a startled newborn, with kindness, 'I see you were startled when Mommy and Daddy yelled and had a fight. Grownups get angry sometimes, especially when we are tired. You're okay, we love you,' mitigates the effect of the fighting." You may think, "How is a newborn going to understand that?" They do! Most of our communication is in the tone of our voice, our body language, and our intention. These are communicated very clearly to your baby. Even though it is true that adult fighting stresses children (even in utero), never feeling angry is an unreasonable expectation for either ourselves or our children. We can notice when we feel angry, own those feelings, and try to talk them out, reassuring the little one that everything is okay.

"The most complex information-processing device ever constructed is on its way," says John Medina, author of *Brain Rules for Baby*. He goes on to say, "During the attachment process, a baby's brain intensely monitors the caregiving it receives. It is essentially asking such things as 'Am I being touched? Am I being fed? Am I safe?' If the baby's requirements are being fulfilled, the brain develops one way; if not, genetic instructions trigger it to develop in another way. It may be a bit disconcerting to realize, but infants have their parents' behaviors in their sights virtually from the moment they come into this world. It is in their evolutionary best interests to do so, of course, which is another way of saying that they can't help it. Babies have nowhere else to turn."

In her book *Philosophical Baby*, Alison Gopnick says, "In adults, vivid awareness accompanies attention, and attention is linked to brain plasticity (the quality of being easily shaped or molded). Attention literally allows us to change our minds and brains. If we made the backwards inference that brain plasticity implies attention, which implies vivid awareness, it would seem that babies are more conscious than we are. They are vividly aware all the time." She concludes that infant awareness is steeped in "a kind of exaltation and a particular kind of happiness."

Once I saw a video of a baby, probably five months old, sitting on a couch with her father on the floor in front of her. He began tearing pieces of paper. She giggled, and then laughed and laughed and laughed, so hard for so long I could hardly believe it. She was the perfect example of this "exaltation and a particular kind of happiness."

In her wonderful book that has yet to be published, *Mothers, Infants and the Evolution of Love*, yoga nun Didi Ananda Uttama writes about how the infant's brain handles stress:

> *As the baby's frontal lobes develop and send out their sinewy fibers, the connections of the stress system grow much stronger and thicker than the calm and connection system. This predisposes him to become a child, and an adult, who's still running on lower brain programming, meaning that he is neurologically primed to trigger a stress response in his brain and body much more easily than a calm or reasoned reaction.*
>
> *Excessive stress responses also pump him up to be less trusting in general, less able to believe that life is on his side. This wiring of joy and intimacy happens not only in the infant but in the mother as well, a significant but often overlooked factor.*

The Development of "Irresistible"

Researchers have speculated over the biological purpose of the joy sparked by an infant in its mother. Uttama has this to say on the subject:

Infant love is a mystery. It brings wonder and awe into the lives of adults, intriguing parents, inspiring poets and stimulating researchers to design ever more sophisticated and subtle means of understanding the minds of our littlest ones. Some theories say that infants, before and after birth, are ensconced in a realm of bliss. There are those that emphasize the sentient qualities of a new being, manifested in the breathtaking sensory and biological developments occurring from the moment of conception. Still others speak intuitively of the spiritual presence of a tiny infant. And some remind us that the entire history of human evolution repeats itself endlessly in the embryonic formation of each new human child. A baby's awareness is being processed by a very down-to-earth, hard-at-work brain adjusting to this new life. A newborn's brain has somewhere around 200 billion brain cells but few synaptic connections. Millions of synapses form during the first years of life, most notably from the last trimester of pregnancy through the second year. There is no other period in life when such a massive proliferation of neuronal connections occurs. The brains of newborns at birth are 25 percent of adult size but grow to 60 percent of adult size by the end of the first year. As a pair of researchers humorously put it, "If the body grew as fast as the brain in the first few years of life, we'd be trying to change the diapers of five- or six-foot-tall toddlers!"

One researcher suggested that this love is a baby's trick of "being irresistible" to make sure that his mother doesn't leave him on the hillside in a fit of desperation. While there may be truth to that, what we cannot resist is a particular kind of subtle, charming state unique to infants and children.

According to the Harvard Center on the Developing Child, in a child's first years of life, seven hundred to one thousand neural connections are formed each second, and by age three, children have approximately 1,000 trillion neuronal connections in their brains. These connections prime them to take in new information, but you have to act fast: after the first few years of life, most of these connections are gradually pruned away.

Neural pathways are a use-it-or-lose-it proposition, so exposing your child to plenty of new foods, languages, and experiences during the first three years of life may shape her into a better-rounded adult and instill good habits early. Humans are calibrated to learn and adapt throughout their lives, but it becomes increasingly difficult to alter the brain's architecture—and the behaviors that result—as time passes and the brain becomes less sensitive to the effects of new experiences. Prolonged stress is toxic to developing brains.

The immaturity of an infant's higher brain (the prefrontal cortex) puts the lower brain (the limbic system and brain stem) in charge by default. This means that fear-driven survival instincts and strong emotions can easily overwhelm the infant and young child with impulses they cannot control. It is the mother's calm, joyous grounding that brings the infant back to balance again and again and again.

"With consistently emotional responsive parenting, the child's frontal lobes will develop essential brain pathways that will, over time, enable him to calm those alarm states in the lower brain," writes Margot Sunderland in her book *The Science of Parenting.* This attention strengthens the circuitry of calm, loving connection and hopefully makes it the default programming. If the nerve fibers connecting the emotional brain with the rational brain are not adequately developed, however, a child can experience feelings of fear or rage and even excessive excitement and not be able to handle the emotions, not knowing how to regulate them appropriately. An overstimulated child throwing a tantrum without caring parental response may well become an out-of-control, angry adult.

John Medina, in his book *Brain Rules for Baby: How to Raise a Smart and Happy Child from Zero to Five,* has a lot to say about brain development:

More than a decade passes between the birth of a baby and its ability to reproduce—an eternity compared with other species. This gap shows not only the depth of the brain's developmental immaturity but also the evolutionary need for unflinchingly attentive parenting. As we evolved, adults who formed protective and continuous teaching relationships with the next generation were at a distinct advantage over those who either could not or would not. In fact, some evolutionary theorists believe that language developed in all its richness just so that this instruction between parent and child could occur with greater depth and efficiency. Relationships among adults were crucial to our survival as well—and they still are, despite ourselves.

He writes that if a baby is "marinated in safety"—that is, in an emotionally stable home—the brain will "cook up beautifully." If not, stress-coping processes fail.

The child is transformed into a state of high alert or a state of complete collapse. If the baby regularly experiences an angry, emotionally violent social environment, his vulnerable little stress responders turn hyperreactive, a condition known as hypercortisolism. If the baby is exposed to severe neglect, like the Romanian orphans, the system becomes underreactive, a condition known as hypocorticolism (hence, the blank stares). Life, to quote Bruce Springsteen, can seem like one long emergency.

Infant Brain Development Is Altered When Parents Argue in Front of Baby

Researchers at the University of Oregon found that babies react to angry, argumentative tones of voice, even while they are asleep. Because infants

are so responsive, severe stresses such as abuse and mistreatment can significantly hamper a baby's brain development. Babies' brains have high
plasticity, which allows them to quickly learn how to respond to the environments and people around them. A number of researchers have investigated how moderate stressors affect babies' brain development.

A 2005 study found that infants' brains devote more attention to angry
voices than happy or neutral tones, and a 2010 study suggested that babies
are attuned to a voice's emotional state. Previous research suggested that
parental conflict can decrease infants' sleep quality and negatively impact
babies' emotional well-being. The researchers presented babies with non-
sense sentences spoken by a male adult voice in a range of emotional
tones—very angry, somewhat upset, neutral, and happy. The results
showed that "even during sleep, infants showed distinct patterns of brain
activity depending on the emotional tone of voice we presented."

Babies' parents completed questionnaires about the level of conflict in
their homes. The brain imaging results indicated that infants from high-
conflict homes showed stronger reactivity to the very angry tone of voice
in brain areas including the hypothalamus, cingulate cortex, caudate nu-
cleus, and thalamus, which are associated with stress and emotional regulation. The research shows that early life experiences can strongly influence
a person's response to events later in life. The results prove that babies are
sensitive to the sounds of parental arguments, though follow-up studies
are necessary to judge the long-term impact of high-conflict homes on
infant brain development. Your baby may not understand exactly what
you're saying, but your tone of voice during arguments is all too clear.

This type of stress shows up behaviorally. Infants whose homes are
unstable are less able to positively respond to new stimuli, calm themselves, and recover from stress; they are unable to regulate their own emotions. Even their extremities sometimes will not develop properly because
stress hormones can interfere with bone mineralization. Newborns can
detect that something is wrong. They can experience physiological
changes—increases in blood pressure, heart rate, and stress hormones—

just like adults. Some researchers claim they can assess the amount of fighting in a marriage simply by taking a twenty-four-hour urine sample from the baby.

If babies do experience this type of stress, Medina says, its effects can be mitigated:

Even infants younger than eight months who are taken from severely traumatized homes and placed in empathic, nurturing environments can show improvements in their stress-hormone regulation in as little as ten weeks. All you have to do is put down the boxing gloves. If marital hostility continues, the children show all the unfortunate behavioral signs of long-term stress. They are at greater risk for anxiety disorders and depression. They catch colds more often, because stress cripples the immune system. They're more antagonistic toward peers. They're less able to focus attention or regulate their emotions. Such children have IQs almost eight points lower than children being raised in stable homes. Predictably, they don't complete high school as often as their peers and attain lower academic achievement when they do.

A baby is sensitive to outside influences even in the womb. Once an infant leaves her comfortable, watery incubator, her brain becomes even more vulnerable. Medina says, "Sustained exposure to hostility can erode a baby's IQ and ability to handle stress, sometimes dramatically. An infant's need for caregiver stability is so strong, he will rewire his developing nervous system depending upon the turbulence he perceives. If you want your child to be equipped with the best brain possible, you need to know about this before you bring home your bundle of joy."

Some stress is normal and even healthy for brains. When a baby is surrounded by supportive adults, the physical effects of stress are usually short-lived and teach them the healthy stress responses they'll need to navigate an unpredictable world. But chronically high stress coupled with a lack of supportive parents can permanently damage neural connections.

It's called "toxic stress," and it can impair health, social skills, and a child's ability to learn.

Maintaining a calm, predictable environment free of extremely stressful conditions such as abuse and mental illness is key. You don't need to shield your child from every little difficulty—the key is to teach kids to cope appropriately when life's road bumps and disappointments arise. And when you can't control the world around you, simply offer your unwavering support—this can be a vital balm in unavoidably high-stress situations.

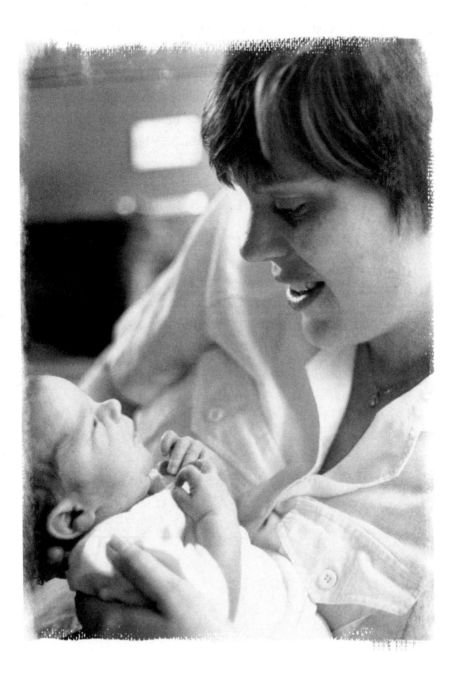

Chapter 11

Music and Massage

Upon what instrument are we two spanned?
And what player has us in his hand?
O sweet song.

—RAINER MARIA RILKE, "LOVESONG"

Music Is Important for Babies

Your voice can be an important part of your baby's massage. By talking softly, humming, or singing, you create an atmosphere of calm. This verbal communication will also help you keep your mind in the present and your attention on your baby.

Singing is a wonderful way to relax. Sing to your baby anytime—while changing diapers, feeding, rocking, or walking. You will discover there are some songs your baby loves to hear again and again. His sense of musical discrimination will astound you.

Familiar lullabies from your own childhood would fit in beautifully here. Think of your grandmother's music box that played a Brahms lullaby or the wonderful, lilting "Alouette" you learned in elementary school. Recall how your own mother sang "Go to Sleep, My Baby" to your younger brother or sisters, and do likewise with your baby.

In one study, parents were asked to sing a song of their choice in two ways. First they were asked to sing as they would to their baby, even though the baby was not present. Then the parent would sing the same song to the baby herself. When other adults were asked to listen to these recordings, they could nearly always identify the song that was sung directly to the infant; these versions tended to be sung at a higher pitch, with much more emotional engagement, elongation of vowel sounds, and more slowly. Interestingly, the fathers sang more slowly to their infants than did the mothers.

This study helps confirm my earlier discussion of how babies respond to their parents' vocalization, when parents unconsciously make it easier for their babies to understand by elongating vowel sounds. So babies actually affect the way parents vocalize; there is a synchrony of interaction that is part of the dance of bonding. Singing is a wonderful way to soothe your baby and capture his attention.

Here are some folk lullabies from around the world. (Notice how most lullabies have many elongated vowel sounds in them). Undoubtedly you have some family favorites to add to this collection. In "References and Recommendations," I have included a list of books and music that will help you utilize this wonderful tool in your practice of infant massage. In addition, the International Association of Infant Massage (the American chapter is called Infant Massage USA) has an online store in which you can purchase several different renditions of our lullaby, "Ami Tomake Bhalobashi Baby." See InfantMassageWarehouse.com and AmiTomake .com.

Lullabies from Around the World

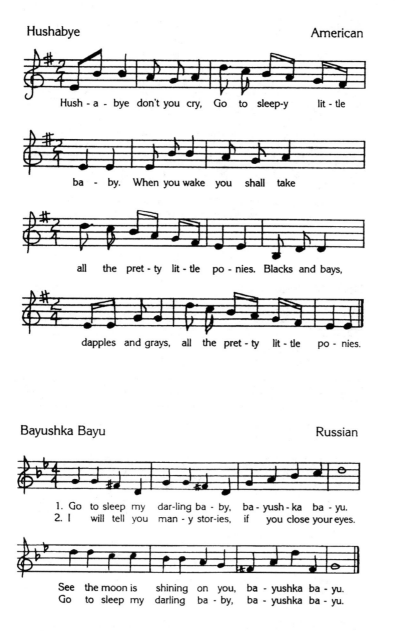

Hushabye — American

Hush - a - bye don't you cry, Go to sleep-y lit - tle
ba - by. When you wake you shall take
all the pret - ty lit - tle po - nies. Blacks and bays,
dapples and grays, all the pret - ty lit - tle po - nies.

Bayushka Bayu — Russian

1. Go to sleep my dar-ling ba - by, ba - yush - ka ba - yu.
2. I will tell you man - y stor-ies, if you close your eyes.

See the moon is shining on you, ba - yushka ba - yu.
Go to sleep my darling ba - by, ba - yushka ba - yu.

Schlaf, Kindlein, Schlaf

German

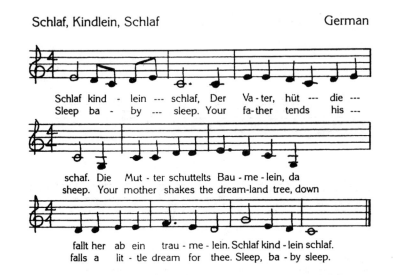

Schlaf kind - lein --- schlaf, Der Va - ter, hüt --- die ---
Sleep ba - by --- sleep. Your fa - ther tends his ---

schaf. Die Mut - ter schuttelts Bau - me - lein, da
sheep. Your mother shakes the dream-land tree, down

fallt her ab ein trau - me - lein. Schlaf kind - lein schlaf.
falls a lit - tle dream for thee. Sleep, ba - by sleep.

Dors, Mon Petit Enfant

French

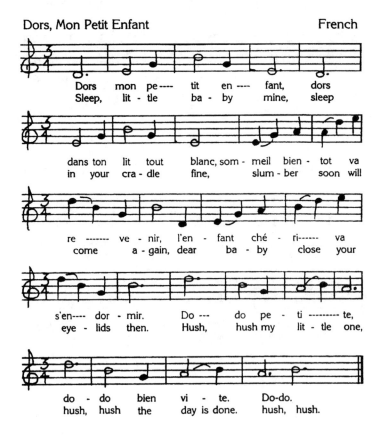

Dors mon pe ---- tit en ---- fant, dors
Sleep, lit - tle ba - by mine, sleep

dans ton lit tout blanc, som - meil bien - tot va
in your cra - dle fine, slum - ber soon will

re ------- ve - nir, l'en - fant ché - ri ------ va
come a - gain, dear ba - by close your

s'en---- dor - mir. Do --- do pe ti --------- te,
eye - lids then. Hush, hush my lit - tle one,

do - do bien vi - te. Do-do.
hush, hush the day is done. hush, hush.

Lullaby — Japanese

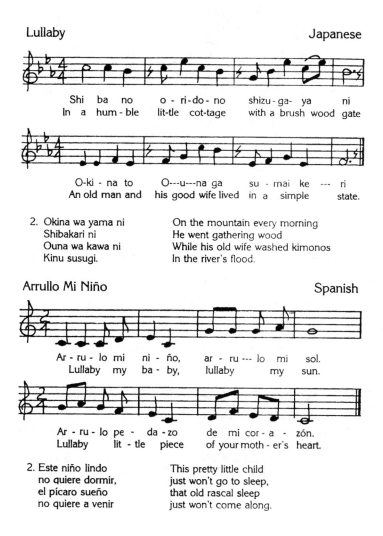

Shi ba no   o - ri-do- no   shizu - ga- ya   ni
In a hum - ble   lit-tle cot-tage   with a brush wood gate

O-ki - na to   O---u---na ga   su - mai ke --- ri
An old man and   his good wife lived in a simple   state.

2. Okina wa yama ni   On the mountain every morning
   Shibakari ni   He went gathering wood
   Ouna wa kawa ni   While his old wife washed kimonos
   Kinu susugi.   In the river's flood.

Arrullo Mi Niño — Spanish

Ar - ru - lo mi   ni - ño,   ar - ru --- lo mi   sol.
Lullaby my   ba - by,   lullaby   my   sun.

Ar - ru - lo pe - da - zo   de mi cor - a - zón.
Lullaby lit - tle piece   of your moth - er's heart.

2. Este niño lindo   This pretty little child
   no quiere dormir,   just won't go to sleep,
   el pícaro sueño   that old rascal sleep
   no quiere a venir   just won't come along.

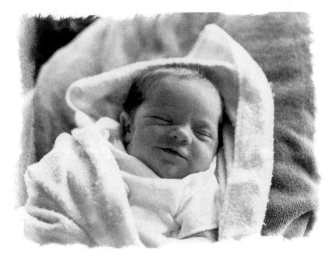

Our Bengali Lullaby

The following Bengali chant from India means "I love you, my dear baby." Its wonderfully soothing effect on babies has made it a favorite in our infant massage classes, and it has become nearly an anthem for the International Association of Infant Massage. The words are pronounced aaah-mee toe-mah-kay, bah-lo-bah-shee baaaabee.

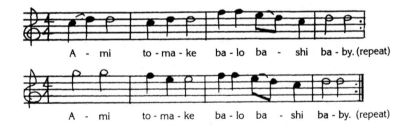

Play Some Music, Tell a Story

If you are not comfortable singing, simply tell a story or talk about the massage as you go. It is the tone of your voice that is most important, not the quality of the words and music you project.

Fathers often find massage time to be a pleasant opportunity to play music they like for background music. Guitar music and pleasant rhythmic tunes that inspire smooth, slow movements seem to work best. Perhaps you have some music in your household that would offer an accompaniment to your baby's massage. A soft symphony, a slow reggae melody, a raga featuring Indian sitar, angelic choir music, or the sound of ocean waves would all provide a beautiful background for your loving touch.

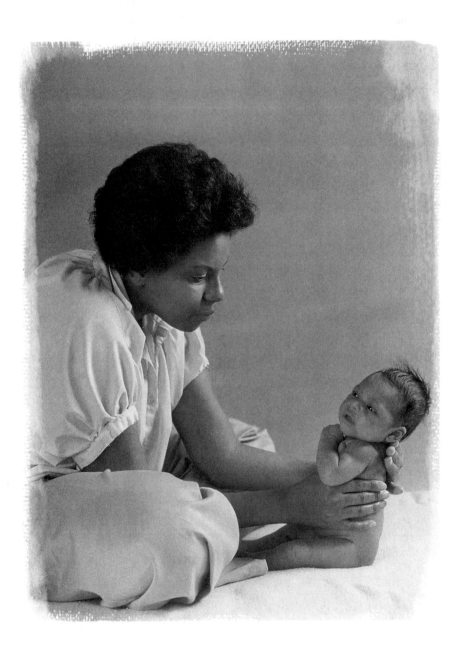

Chapter 12

Getting Ready

O young thing, your mother's lovely armful!
How sweet the fragrance of your body!

—EURIPIDES

Start as Soon as You Wish

Even without conscious awareness, a mother will usually begin massaging her baby, ever so gently, from the moment of birth. It is a part of the bonding process—a biological urge to know her baby through all her senses.

The massage in this book can be started as soon as you desire. For the first six or seven months, your baby will benefit most from a daily massage. As your child becomes more active through crawling or walking, you may reduce it to once a week, as desired. Your toddler may enjoy a rubdown before bed or after bath time. In this case, you should certainly continue it. In Chapter 18 we will discuss what modifications you will need to make for your child's larger body and different needs. Here I'll tell you about some of the things you might want to set up before you begin.

Massage Oil

As your hands glide over your baby's delicate skin, the last thing you want to do is to create any sort of friction. You will need a light natural oil to work with. The only exception to this might be when baby's skin is very dry, in which case an oil-based lotion that absorbs into the skin may help soften even more. But for regular massages, oil is better than lotion because lotions tend to soak into the skin quite rapidly, which means you would constantly have to stop the massage in order to reapply it.

The primary benefit of oil is that it makes the movement smoother on the baby's skin. As you are working, you apply the oil to your hands; use a quarter-size amount to begin with.

For a number of reasons, I prefer cold-pressed fruit and/or vegetable oils, and stay completely away from the mass-produced, heavily advertised "baby oils." From my research in this area, I have developed the belief that a significant amount of what we put on our skin is absorbed deep within the body. If such is the case, then we quite naturally want to try to nourish our little ones topically, and not use a product that may actually rob them of vital nutrients.

Mass-produced "baby oils" have a nonorganic, nonfood petroleum base. Their primary ingredient is mineral oil. To get mineral oil, gasoline and kerosene are removed from the crude petroleum by heating, in a method called fractional distillation. By using sulfuric acid, applying absorbents, and washing with solvents and alkalis, hydrocarbons and other chemicals are then removed.

Not only is there no food value in this type of oil, but such a product may actually deplete the system of a number of nutrients, including vitamins A, D, E, and K. Some authorities, such as Adelle Davis, believe that mineral oil, when ingested, produces deficiencies of the vitamins listed, and specifically recommend against its use as a baby oil. When you're in the middle of a massage and baby touches herself and then puts her hand in or near her mouth, you don't want to worry that such a nonfood substance is passing into her delicate digestive system.

Infants, whose brains and nervous systems are not fully developed, are particularly vulnerable to substances absorbed by the skin. Commercially produced mineral oils also dry the skin and clog its pores. Most modern pediatricians discourage their use for this reason alone. These oils were not made for massage, which encourages the absorption of whatever substance you are using. That substance, in my view, should be a food product that nourishes the skin. I also stay away from those that have an alcohol base, because they are drying and may cause skin reactions.

If the oil you select is enhanced with vitamin E, so much the better, since this vitamin has been shown to be especially healing to the skin. It is also a natural antioxidant, which means that it inhibits rancidity. Cold-pressed oils keep the natural vitamin E intact; refining through heating or other procedures tends to destroy it.

Odor is an often overlooked part of the bonding process. An infant's olfactory system is ready to function as early as seventeen weeks gestation, so it must be an important function for the newborn. A highly refined sense of smell immediately following birth helps a baby distinguish his mother's chemical "signature." Unfortunately, we often assault our infants' senses with noxious smells and thus inhibit this means of bonding. For this reason, I recommend that you use an unscented oil for your newborn's massage. (In the "Resources" section, I list recommended sources for baby massage oils.) Regular bathing keeps baby's pores from clogging and rashes from developing. As a test, you may first want to apply your oil to a patch of your baby's skin, and leave it for a couple of hours, to make sure she isn't allergic to, for example, a nut oil.

Time and Place

You will want to experiment to discover the times and place that are best for you and your baby. Generally, morning is a good time to begin, when both of you have been fed and are ready for the day. However, there are also advantages to afternoon and evening massages. For some babies, a

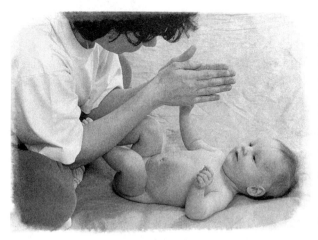

massage before a bath and then a nap is good for releasing that last bit of energy so they can sleep more soundly. For others, however, there is a point of no return, when any stimulation is too much and all the baby needs is rest. In this case, give the massage right after the nap.

Evening is also a good time for some; if baby is tired but not too cranky, it might also help him to sleep. Your schedule must also be considered. You may work outside the home or have other small children to care for. Evening may be the best time for you, when the day's work is done and the baby's other parent can watch the other children for a few minutes. A massage gives you and your newborn the time together that you both deserve.

In the early months, a delightful routine is to massage the baby, then fill a warm bath and take her in with you. The bath becomes a wonderfully relaxing experience, and your baby may even fall asleep in your arms. To her, the experience is rather like a "womb with a view," in that she floats in the womblike warm water, yet, at the same time, sees you as you support her with comfort and security. She may cry when you take her out of the tub, but usually some cuddling and/or nursing will quiet her.

You're probably wondering how both of you can get out of the tub safely and without becoming chilled. First, be sure the bathroom is nice and warm. Keep an infant seat covered with towels next to the tub, and when you are ready to get out, put her in the seat, swaddling her with towels. Then you can get out and dry off, and perhaps you can both crawl into bed for a nap, or get going with your day.

From about six months of age, when bath time becomes more of a playtime for your baby, the massage works better later in the day, when she is a little more tired and is almost ready for a nap. The massage can help her release that last bit of tension so she can sleep deeply.

Warmth

Always massage in a warm, quiet place. If you feel a little too warm, it is probably the right temperature for infant massage. Peter Wolff, a well-known pediatrician and researcher who completed countless studies of newborns and their behavior, observed that temperature has an important effect on the amount of time babies sleep and on their crying. Babies kept at warmer temperatures, he found, cried less and slept more than those subjected to cooler environments.

Rudolf Steiner, philosopher, scientist, educator, and propounder of Waldorf Education, also stressed the importance of keeping babies warm. He asserted that the formative forces, both physical and spiritual, that work to help babies' bodies and souls grow properly need this warmth to be effective.

I have observed that babies in our infant massage classes, especially those under three months of age, are much more comfortable, startle less, and relax more easily if they are kept quite warm. If your room is cool, you may want to place a small, safe portable heater in the room. Or you can wrap a baby-size warm-water bottle in a towel and tuck it under the blanket near the baby's feet for the massage. The room should be warm enough so that you can wear light clothing and still feel warm. Remember, your baby has much less bulk to keep him warm, and without clothing he could be chilled, which can cause fussing.

Ideally, your baby is naked for the massage, so you can move smoothly through the strokes, which helps integrate the baby's limbs with his torso. You may want to place a cloth over his genitals to prevent accidents. Turn off cellphones, TVs, and computers nearby. Focus just on your baby with as few interruptions as possible.

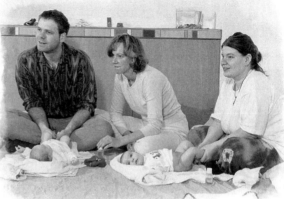

Positioning

Find a comfortable sitting position for massaging your baby. Your back should be relatively straight, with most of your movement coming from your lower back as a center. You can sit on the floor or on a bed cross-legged with your baby in front of you on a pillow or blanket covered with a towel; some baby-care companies even make pillows especially for this purpose. Remember to bring the baby as close to you as possible, with his bottom firmly resting against your crossed legs.

Cradle Pose

During the newborn period, the position used in India, which I call the Cradle Pose, can work wonderfully if your body can do it without discomfort. Here's how: Sit on the floor with legs stretched out, back supported against a wall or furniture. Now bend your knees slightly outward, touching the soles of your feet together slightly. Pad the area between your knees with thick, towel-covered blankets, making an indentation in the middle for your baby. Place the baby in the "cradle" of your legs, facing you. This position helps the baby feel more securely positioned and helps conserve warmth. Because babies have the tonic neck reflex for the first four to six months, it is natural for them to look off to the side when lying flat; the angle of your legs in Cradle Pose helps tip the baby up slightly toward you, and placing the baby's head at the arches of your feet will help keep his head aligned for eye contact.

You can give a massage in other positions as well. You can use a changing table, all the better if the table can be lowered so you can sit in a chair and relax. Using a changing table is a last resort, however; the baby probably isn't facing you, and if you have to stand up, you can't relax as much as you should or be physically close enough to your newborn. Massage can be given in sections and at various times. After changing the diaper, you can massage your baby's legs, arms, or back, and use Touch Relaxation and Resting Hands to reinforce your regular massage sessions.

The Massage Technique: How Much Pressure?

Infant massage is not manipulative in the way adult massage by a professional massage therapist may be; there is no vigorous kneading or chopping. It is a gentle, firm, warm communication. A baby's muscles, which make up only a quarter of his total body weight (as compared to almost half in adulthood), aren't developed enough to have knots of tension. His body is so tiny that a gentle but firm stroke is enough to stimulate circulation and tone the internal functions.

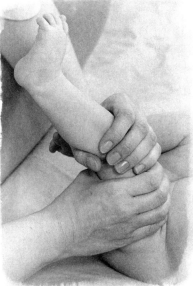

In the beginning, while you are learning and your baby is tiny, be soft and gentle. As your baby grows, your massage will grow firmer. Do not be afraid to touch her firmly. You will find she enjoys being handled and massaged in a manner that communicates your strength, love, and confidence. All of your strokes should be comfortable but stimulating. Avoid stroking your baby with a fluttery, poking, or tickling touch. The massage given here should be done as much as possible with your whole hand molding to the baby's body with a gentle but firm pressure, just enough to encourage circulation and let your baby know she is in the hands of a strong, capable parent.

Infants Are Sensitive to Pleasant Touch

Cognitive neuroscientist Merle Fairhurst and colleagues at the Max Planck Institute for Human Cognitive and Brain Sciences in Leipzig, Germany, knew that previous studies with adults show that a specific type of touch receptor is activated in response to a particular stroking velocity, leading to the sensation of "pleasant touch." They hypothesized that this type of response might emerge as early as infancy.

Babies show unique physiological and behavioral responses to pleasant touch, which helps to cement the bonds between parent and child. For this study, Fairhurst and colleagues had infants sit in their parents' laps while the experimenter stroked the back of the infant's arm with a paintbrush. The results showed that the babies' heart rate slowed in response to the brushstrokes when the strokes were of medium velocity; in other words, this kind of touch helped to decrease their physiological arousal.

The infant's slower heart rate during medium-velocity brushstrokes was uniquely correlated with the parent's own self-reported sensitivity to touch. The more sensitive the parent was to touch, the more the infant's heart rate slowed in response to medium-velocity touch.

This study indicates that a baby who is massaged regularly, receiving pleasant touch, will experience bonding, and is therefore more likely to naturally bond with his/her own children later in life. It also reminds us to do the strokes in a way that is equivalent to "medium velocity"—that is, not too light, not too firm. In my experience, most parents err on the side of too light a stroke and often need to be encouraged to be a little more firm as they massage. When they know that their baby responds better to a firmer stroke, they gain confidence. I often asked them to think of a cat licking her kittens; the "stroke" is just right, and the kittens rely on the mother's strength to feel grounded and cared for.

How to Begin

Assemble massage oil, towels, a few extra diapers, and a change of clothes for baby. You should wear something comfortable that you wouldn't mind getting a little soiled. Before beginning, warm the area, wash your hands, remove your jewelry, and relax your body. Take a few minutes to sit quietly, with your eyes closed or looking at your baby. Starting at the top of your head, relax every muscle in your body as much as you can.

Breathe in fully, then breathe out as you slowly drop your head forward; breathe in and out, then in again, as you raise your head to neutral, and breathe out. You will feel a pull on the back of your neck, shoulders, and upper back. Repeat this again to fully relax yourself. Feel the relaxation wash over you.

Now take three more breaths. With the first breath, affirm: "I now let go of all tension. My body is relaxed." Feel all traces of tension or anxiety leave your body. You are confident and centered.

With the second breath, affirm: "I release all other thoughts and focus on my baby." Let all worries and plans leave your mind, like birds flying through a clear blue sky. You are here now—just you and your baby. You deserve this time together.

With the third breath, affirm: "I am the gentle power of love, flowing through my hands to my baby." Visualize all the love you feel for your baby as a brilliant sun in the center of your heart. With each heartbeat, its warm radiance courses through your arms, into your hands, and over your baby as you begin the massage.

A harmonious mind parallels slow, deep, and regular breathing. As you massage your baby, breathe deeply and slowly so that your lungs fill with air down into your belly, and then exhale completely. Once in a while, make an audible sigh, breathing in through your nose and exhaling through your mouth, at the same time as you consciously relax your body. Your baby will feel this and begin to imitate your relaxing sighs. You are now ready to begin the massage.

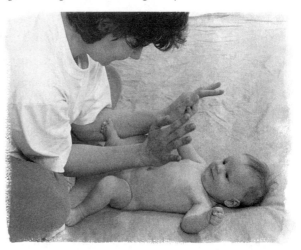

Request Permission to Begin

If this is your first session, you may want to remove just the bottom half of your baby's clothing, as I encourage you to begin with only the legs today. Do remove the diaper, though, and lightly cover the front with a loose cloth or diaper to protect yourself from mishaps. In subsequent sessions, you can begin to add more strokes. It may take a few or many sessions before your baby enjoys a full body massage. You will know as you go along how much massage the baby wants and needs as you get to know the routine and your baby becomes comfortable with it. Remove all of your baby's clothing as soon as you can.

- As you remove his clothing, tell him that it is massage time.
- Pour a small amount of massage oil into your palm. Now rub your palms together to warm them, saying, "It's time for massage." Your baby will hear the oil swishing between your hands and alert to the sound of the word *massage*.
- Show your palms to your baby, saying, "May I massage you now?" The first time, of course, your baby doesn't know what is about to happen. But in subsequent sessions, this routine will become a cue to which he will respond.

How can you tell if your baby is saying no? Usually the baby will make disengaging cues, such as throwing his hands up in a guarding motion, turning his head away, kicking, and fussing. The baby may begin to hiccup, flail his arms, and move his eyes around frantically.

If you get a no, you may want to try warming up the space or covering him with a blanket, bring him closer to you, and lay your warm hands on his legs, using deep relaxation—the Resting Hands we talked about in Chapter 9. Then ask again. Often a small change in comfort is all that is necessary. Or maybe you need to relax more deeply. Think of things you could do to change the atmosphere to make it more warm and comfortable for your baby.

If you still get a very clear no, wait for another time to try again. If the baby seems a little fussy but not definite, continue the massage. Often a fussy baby will calm down and start enjoying the massage after you have finished one or both legs. The next time you massage, the experience will be more familiar, and the fussing should diminish.

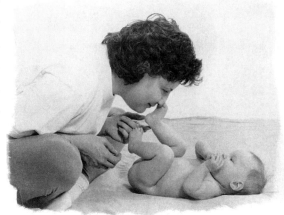

This preparatory routine serves several important purposes. It lets the baby know that a new experience is about to begin, and it helps him to get ready for it. It also communicates—through your voice and your body language—respect for him. It says, "You are worthy of respect. You are in charge of your body, and people should ask your permission to interact with you in this way." Later, in Chapter 18, we will discuss how these early experiences can help your child know the difference between healthy and unhealthy touching as he grows older. Using these cues before beginning a massage now will help build the trust, respect, and values that will ensure a healthy life.

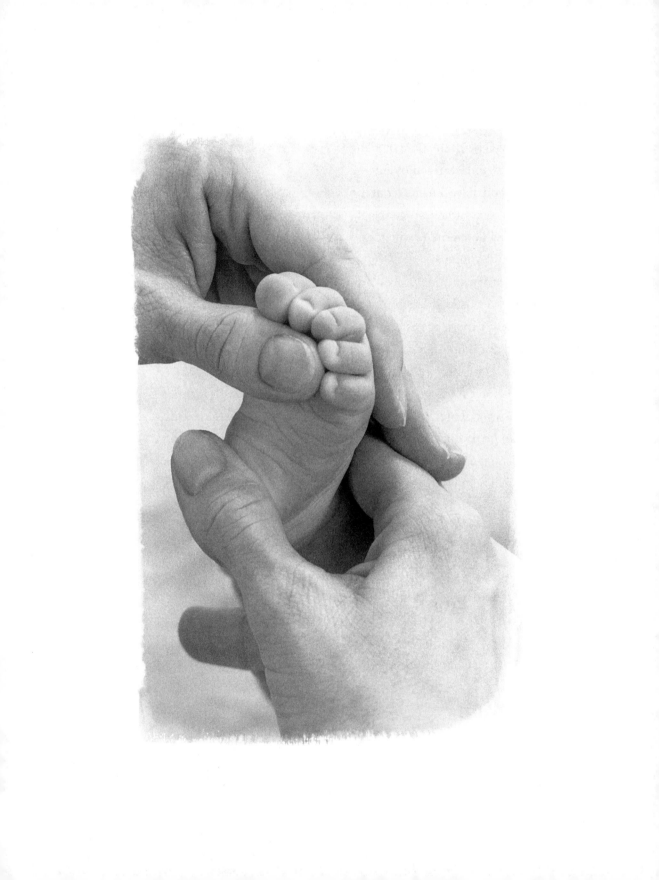

Chapter 13

How to Massage Your Baby

When from the wearying war of life
I seek release
I look into my baby's face
And there find peace.

—MARTHA FOOTE CROW, "PEACE"

Just the Two of You

As you massage your baby, every movement of your body will be an expression of your love. Your strong but gentle touch, the rhythm you create, the way you move back and forth with each stroke, your eyes, your smile, and your voice are all as much a part of the experience as the massage itself. Gaze into your baby's eyes and open yourself to the love you share. Relax, and begin your massage by making gentle contact with your baby's skin. Feel your hands, heavy, warm, and relaxed, supporting your baby. Unless otherwise indicated, repeat each stroke at least three or four times.

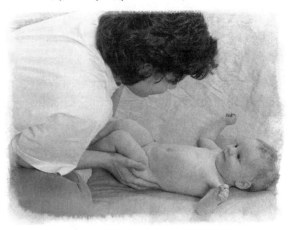

The Order of Strokes Is Important

Originally, the Indian massage started with the chest. I discovered that starting with the legs and feet is much better. Babies reach out to the world with their legs and feet. Observe your baby closely when interacting with new people. Before making eye contact, most infants will wiggle their feet and legs. You may detect a kind of sign language your baby uses with her feet to make contact with other people and establish trust. Even two babies brought into proximity will kick and wiggle their legs, as if conversing with each other with their feet!

The feet and legs are the least vulnerable part of your baby's body. If, right at first, you begin massaging her torso, she may become tense and anxious. She will instinctively "close" her arms and legs to protect her vital organs. Beginning with the legs and feet gives her a chance to establish trust and accept the massage gradually. For many babies, massage of the legs and feet is also the most pleasurable part of the experience. Thus, beginning with the legs will help baby to relax all over.

Sensitive Areas

If your baby has been hospitalized for any reason, she probably received heel sticks when hospital personnel drew blood for testing. Sensitivity in this area can remain long after the bruises have disappeared. If your baby seems to react with fear or displeasure when you begin to massage her foot, stop using the strokes and simply hold her foot gently in your palms, molding your hands to it. Use Resting Hands for a few days to help her accept touch, then try stroking again.

This sensitivity may happen in other areas as well: a baby with gastro-intestinal difficulties will react when you massage her tummy, a baby who has had heart-monitor pads stuck to her chest will react to the chest massage, and most newborns instinctively hold their arms close as they did in the womb. Using Resting Hands, gently shake, pat, and say, "Ree-laaxx . . ." And then give her positive feedback when she lets go.

"May I Massage Your Legs and Feet?"

The Indian and Swedish Milking strokes aid circulation to the feet and back toward the heart. The Hug and Glide stroke and the Rolling stroke help tone and relax the legs. Massage one leg and foot, and then the other.

1. INDIAN MILKING

Milk the leg with the inside edge of each hand, encompassing the leg and molding your hands to it, one following the other. The opposite hand gently holds the ankle. The outside hand should move over the buttock; the inside hand moves inside the thigh and up the leg to the ankle.

Move in rhythmic strokes, with your lower back/pelvis as your center of gravity. Remember to use the bottom hand to keep your baby's pelvis on the floor, so that you do not lift the baby's body with your strokes.

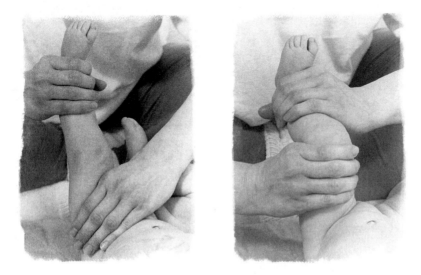

2. HUG AND GLIDE

Hold the leg with the inside edge of your hands facing upward. Keep your hands together so as not to twist the knee joint, and encompass the leg as much as possible. Stroke from the thigh to the ankle, gently turning your hands in opposite directions, forward and back, squeezing very gently. This stroke moves across the muscle and thus helps it relax.

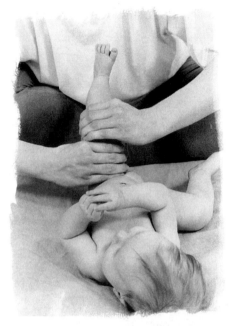

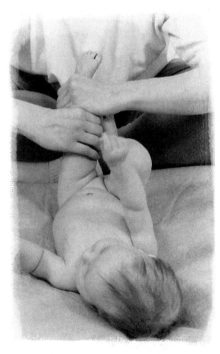

3. THUMB OVER THUMB

Stroke your thumbs, one after the other, from the heel to the toes.

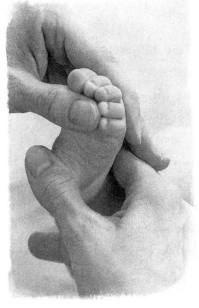

4. TOE ROLL

Squeeze and roll each toe.

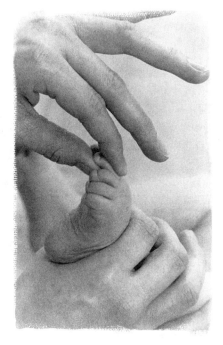

The Foot

There are seventy-two thousand nerve endings in each foot. The many theories of how foot massage works all agree that points on the feet connect with other body areas. Environmental stresses can cause imbalances in our system that we experience as colds, flu, ear infections, and so on. Reflexologists (those who study and work with these points on the feet) say that by-products of these imbalances, uric acid and excess calcium, can calcify around nerve endings in the feet, blocking the flow of energy through the body. Foot massage, they say, moves the excess calcium and uric acid out, so that they are absorbed by the blood and lymph and eventually excreted out of the body.

5. UNDER TOES
With your forefinger, gently press the ball of the foot, just under the toes.

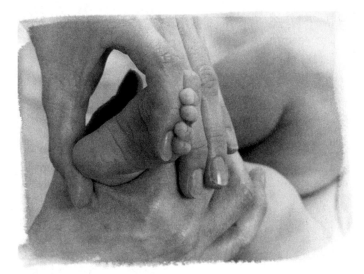

6. HEEL OF FOOT

With your forefinger, press the ball of the foot where the heel begins, and massage this area gently.

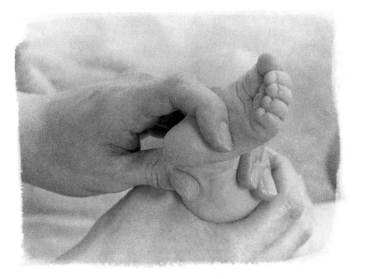

7. THUMB PRESS

Press in with your thumbs all over the bottom of the foot.

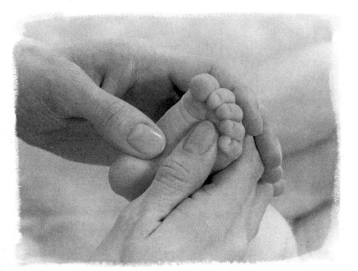

8. TOP OF FOOT

Using your thumbs, one after the other, stroke the top of the foot toward the ankle.

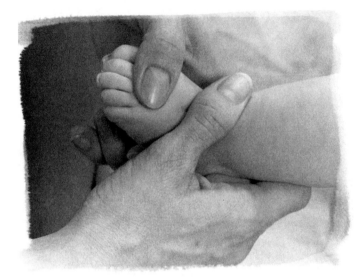

9. ANKLE CIRCLES

Make small circles all around the ankle with your thumbs.

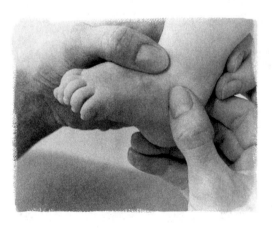
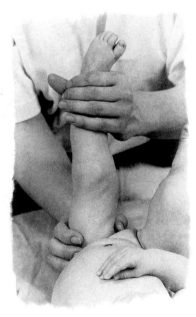

10. SWEDISH MILKING

Milk the leg from ankle to hip, stabilizing the leg at the ankle, moving one hand on the outside of the leg, then the other on the inside. Remember not to pull the baby's body up off the surface.

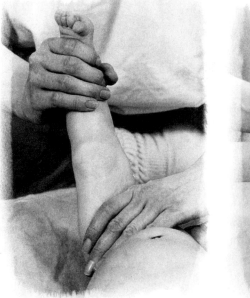
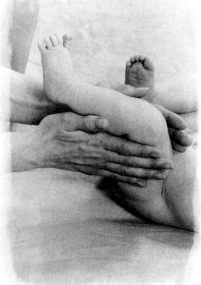

11. ROLLING

Roll the leg between your hands from thigh to ankle. Most babies love this!

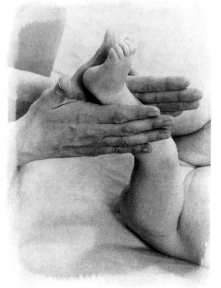

12. BOTTOM RELAXER

After massaging each leg and foot, massage the buttocks with both hands in small circles, then stroke the legs to the feet, gently bouncing.

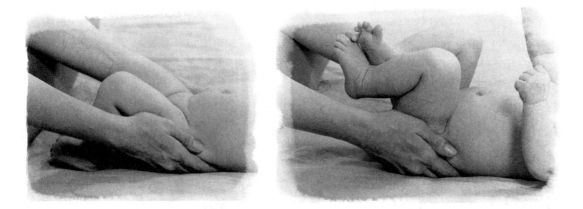

13. INTEGRATION

Move both hands with a sweeping stroke from buttocks to feet. This integrates the legs with the torso and lets baby know you are moving to another part of the body.

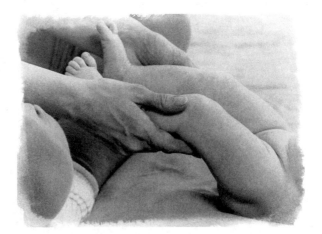

"May I Massage Your Tummy?"

The strokes for the stomach will tone your baby's intestinal system and help relieve gas and constipation. Most of the strokes end at the baby's lower left belly (your right). This is where the eliminative part of the intestine is located. The purpose is to move gas and intestinal matter toward the bowel. Always stroke from the rib cage down, and use a clockwise motion for circular strokes. If you have a colicky baby, a special routine is given in Chapter 15.

1. RESTING HANDS

Start by making contact with your baby's tummy, laying your hand on the belly with a heavy, warm, relaxed feeling, letting your baby know it is time to massage the belly.

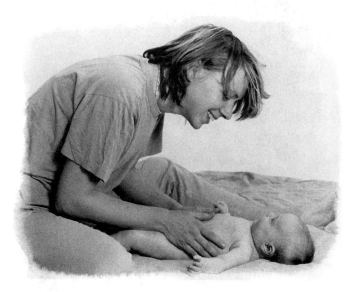

2. WATER WHEEL PART A

Make paddling strokes on your baby's tummy, one hand following the other, as if you were scooping a depression into sand. Keep your hands molded to the baby's tummy. Do not use the edge of your hand. Repeat about six times.

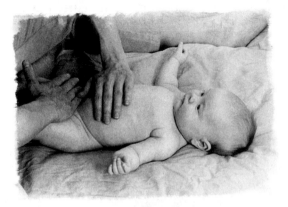

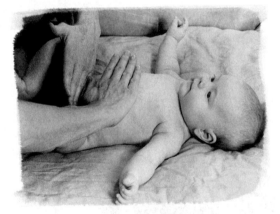

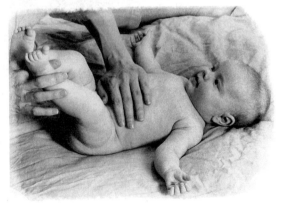

3. WATER WHEEL PART B

Hold your baby's legs up with one hand, grasping the ankles gently. Your baby's body should be close to you, hips anchored firmly on the floor. Do not lift the baby's body. With your other hand, repeat the paddling motion. This will relax the stomach and permit you to extend the massage a little more deeply.

Another way to hold your baby's legs up for this stroke is to cross your left hand under the baby's right leg and hold on to the left, so your left arm holds up both legs. Stroke with the right hand. (You can reverse this if your dominant hand is the left.)

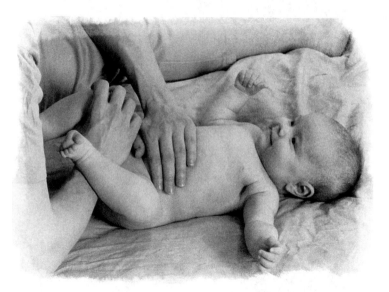

4. THUMBS TO SIDES

With thumbs flat at the baby's navel, push out to the sides. Be sure you use the flat thumbs, and do not poke.

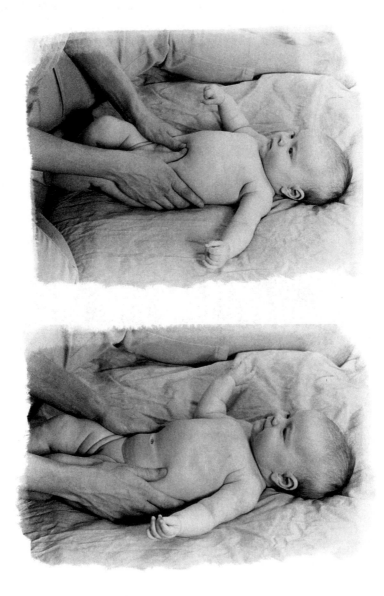

5. SUN MOON

Your left hand strokes in a full circle, moving clockwise starting at your left (seven o'clock). As the left hand is making the lower part of the circle, the right hand makes a half moon above, just below the rib cage, stroking from baby's right to left (your left to right), like an upside-down U.

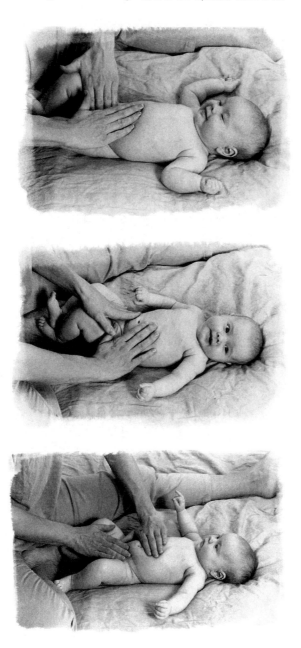

6. I LOVE YOU

As you go through this series of strokes, say "I—love—youuuu!" in a high-pitched, cooing tone. Your baby will love it! First, make a single I-shaped stroke with your right hand on baby's left belly several times, pressing the pads of your fingers straight down from baby's rib cage as you say, "*Iiiiiii.*"

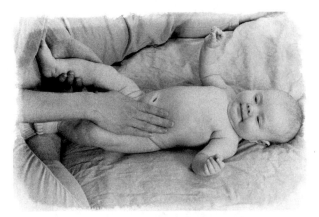

Next, make a backward, sideways L going from your left to right and then down, as you say "*looooooooove.*"

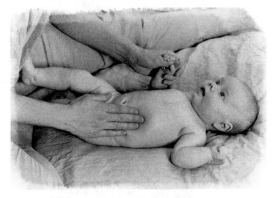

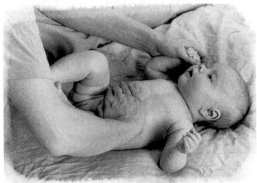

Make an upside-down U, going from your left to right (from baby's right to left), with the upper part of the stroke under the rib cage, as you say "yooooooooou."

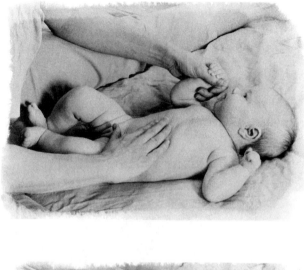

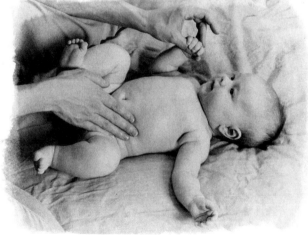

7. WALKING

Using the flat part of your fingers, walk across your baby's tummy at the navel, from your left to right. You may feel some gas bubbles moving under your fingers. After massaging the tummy, move smoothly into the chest strokes.

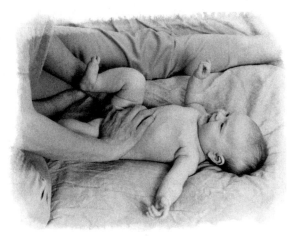

"May I Massage Your Chest?"

Massaging the chest helps tone the lungs and the heart. Imagine that you are freeing the baby's breath and filling her heart with love. Begin by greeting the baby's chest with Resting Hands.

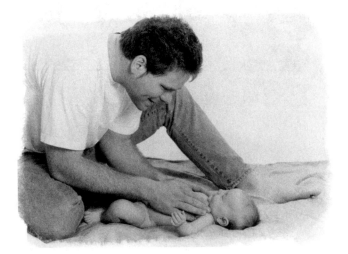

1. OPEN BOOK

With both hands together at the center of the chest, stroke out to the sides, following the rib cage, as if you were flattening the pages of a book. Keep your hands in contact with your baby as you move them down, around, and up to your starting point, similar to a heart-shaped motion. The pressure is from the center outward; the rest is just to keep hands in contact with the body.

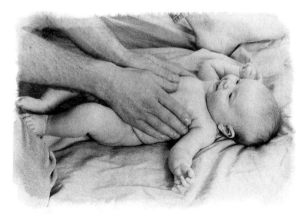

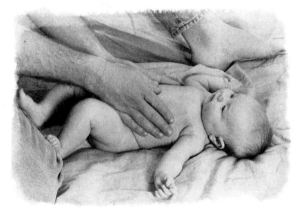

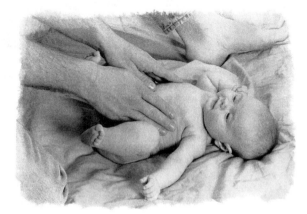

2. BUTTERFLY

To begin this stroke, both hands mold to the baby's rib cage.

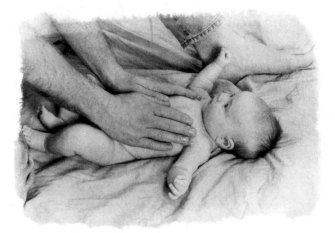

The right hand moves across the chest diagonally, to the baby's right shoulder. Then, pulling gently at the shoulder, the hand moves back diagonally to the rib cage. Be careful not to nick the baby's chin with your fingernails.

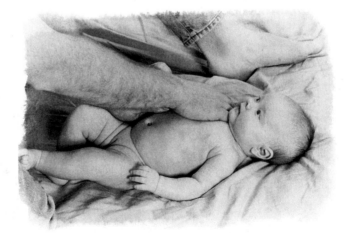

Now the left hand moves across the chest diagonally, to the baby's left shoulder, repeating the same motion. Follow one hand with the other, rhythmically crisscrossing the chest. There is more pressure on the forward motion than coming back. Remember to move from your center of gravity— your lower back—keeping your arms and hands relaxed and warm.

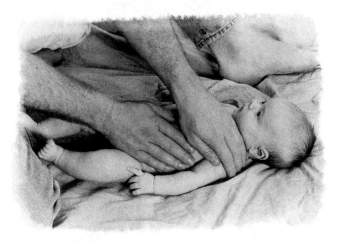

3. INTEGRATION

Sweep both hands from chest to tummy, all the way to the feet, to integrate all of the strokes you have just performed.

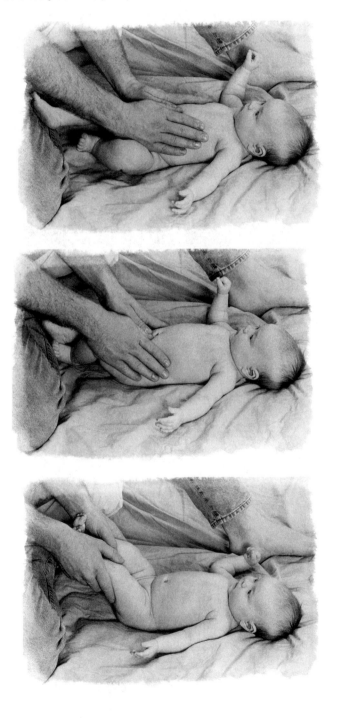

"May I Massage Your Arms and Hands?"

When massaging the arms, the complementary differences between Swedish and Indian methods are strikingly revealed in the Milking motions. We use both methods, combining the Indian concept of balancing and releasing tension with the muscle-toning Swedish massage to promote circulation.

1. RESTING HANDS

Start by greeting your baby's arms with warm, gentle touch and requesting permission.

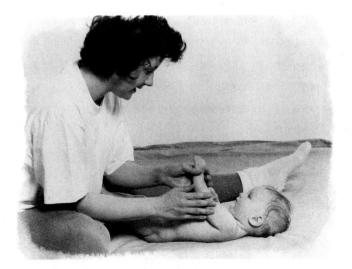

2. PIT STOP

First stroke the armpit a few times, massaging the important lymph nodes in that area.

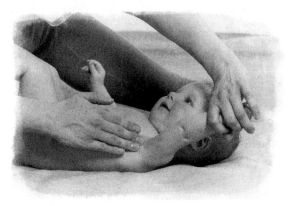

Some babies resist having their arms massaged and will protectively hug their arms close to their chest. In this case, rather than pulling outward on your baby's arm, massage it toward the direction she is holding it. Support her in protecting herself, massaging the arm in its "hug" position. When she begins to feel relaxed and supported, she will begin to relax her arms and "give" them to you for massage.

This photo shows the Indian Milking stroke being done with the baby holding her arm in tight. The parent supports her in that, just massaging in the way that she can in this position. Usually then the baby will begin to open up.

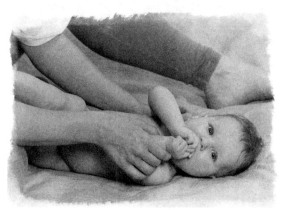

3. INDIAN MILKING

Holding your baby's wrist with your hand, milk the arm with the other hand, starting at the shoulder and moving to the wrist. Immediately follow with your other hand, one hand after the other. Use the inside of your hand, molding it as much as possible to the baby's arm.

For tiny babies, you may start just using three fingers; eventually you can use your whole hand in a warm, encompassing stroke. Stabilize the baby's shoulder so as not to pull the body up off the surface.

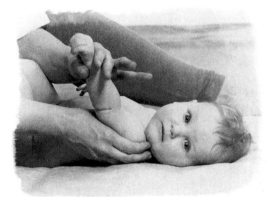

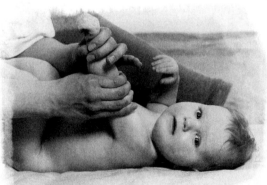

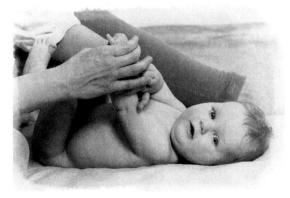

4. HUG AND GLIDE

Hold your hands together around the baby's arm, then gently move your hands in opposite directions, keeping your hands together so as not to twist the elbow joint. With this stroke, you are gently massaging across the muscle, encouraging it to relax.

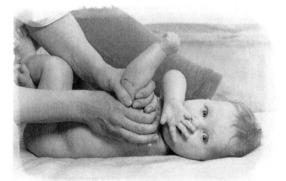

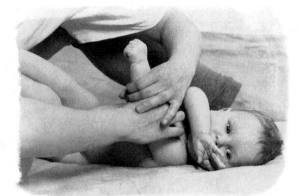

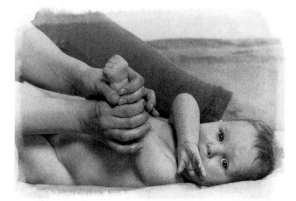

5. FINGER ROLL

Open your baby's hand with your thumbs, and roll each finger between your index finger and thumb.

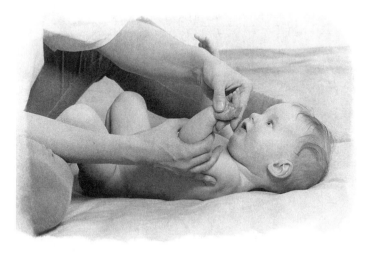

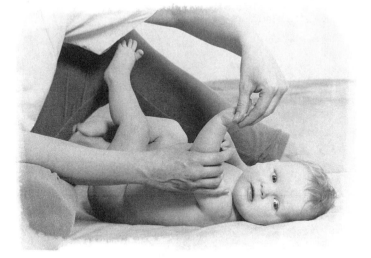

6. TOP OF HAND

Stroke the top of the hand.

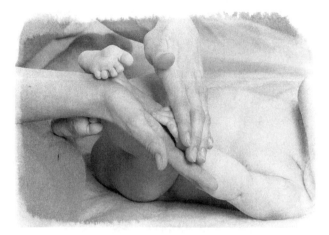

7. WRIST CIRCLES

Massage the wrist, making small circles all around.

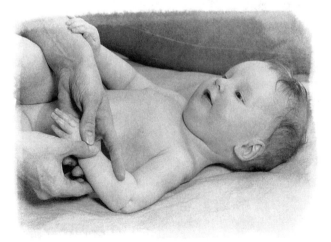

8. SWEDISH MILKING

Milk the arm from the wrist to the shoulder, one hand following the other. Just as in Indian Milking, try to mold your hand to the baby's arm. Stabilize your baby's shoulder so as not to pull the body up. Again, with tiny babies, you may use only three fingers to do this stroke at first.

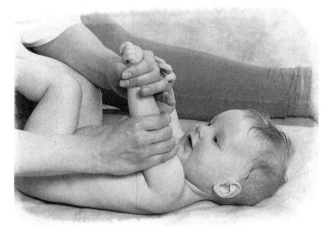

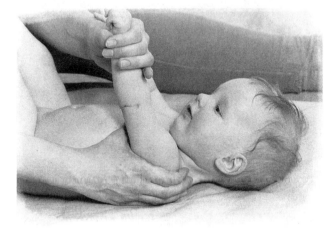

9. ROLLING

Roll your baby's arm between your hands from shoulder to wrist, several times. This is a fun and relaxing stroke for babies of any age!

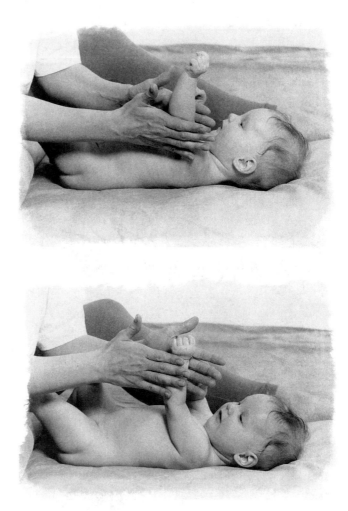

10. TOUCH RELAXATION

Use Touch Relaxation to help your baby relax and release her arm. Gently mold your hands to the baby's arm, letting your hands feel heavy and relaxed. Use your voice, saying "Reee-laaaxx" or "Let go" as you gently pat, roll, and bounce the arm to encourage muscle relaxation. When you feel the muscles relax, give your baby positive feedback: "Very good! You relaxed your arm!"

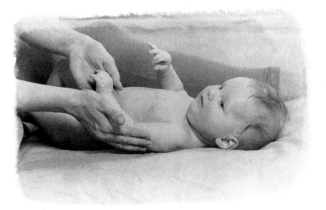

11. INTEGRATION

Sweep your hands from baby's shoulders to chest, tummy, legs, and feet in a single stroke, integrating the whole body.

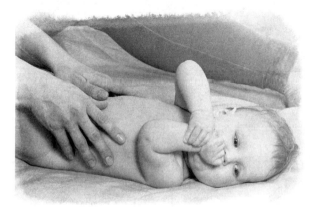

"May I Massage Your Face?"

A baby's face accumulates a lot of tension by sucking, teething, crying, and generally interacting with the world around her. I am often asked why I do not include strokes for the head here, and focus instead on the face. There are several reasons. First, many infants' heads are sensitive, their bones still moving and growing as the plates shift and the soft spot hardens. Second, massaging the head can cause memories of the difficulty of pushing out of the birth canal, and so birth-trauma-type crying can ensue. In addition, there is no real musculature in the head that needs relaxing at this point. When your baby is four to six months old and you are very familiar with the massage, try cupping baby's head and making small circles, to see if she likes it or not. If so, you can include it in your routine at this point.

1. OPEN BOOK

Using the flat part of your fingers, start at the middle of the forehead and stroke out to the sides, as if flattening the pages of a book, moving your hands down along the sides of the face. Try not to cover your baby's eyes and nose with your hands.

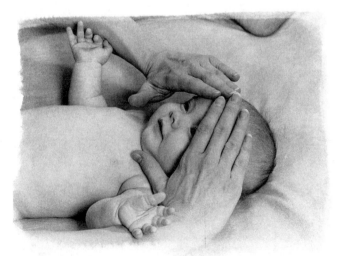

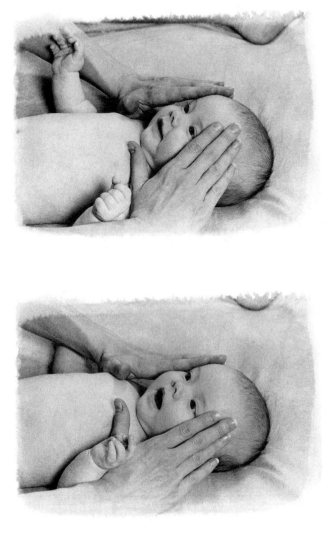

2. RELAX YOUR EYES

With your thumbs, stroke lightly over the eyebrows from the center outward.

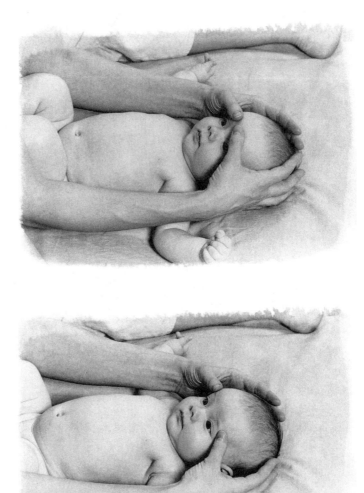

3. HAPPY SINUSES AND CHEEK MUSCLES

With your thumbs, push up on the bridge of the nose, then stroke down diagonally across the cheeks. This helps open the sinuses and relax the cheek muscles.

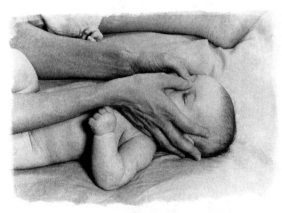

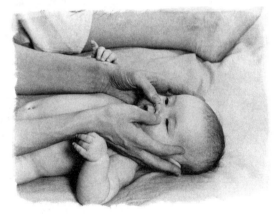

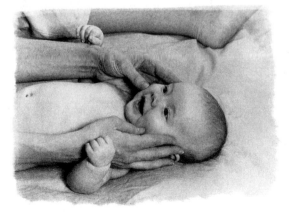

4. SMILE

With your thumbs, make a smile first on the upper lip, then on the lower lip.

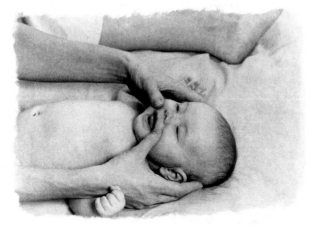

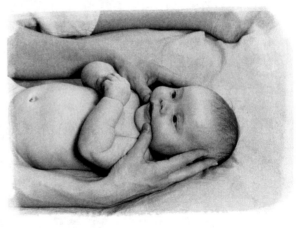

5. RELAX THE JAW

Make small circles around the jaw with your fingertips.

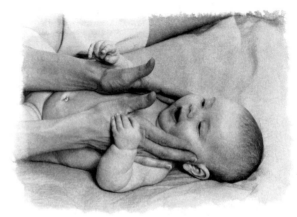

6. EARS, NECK, AND ALL OF THOSE CHINS!

Using the fingertips of both hands, stroke over the ears, around the back of the ears, and pull up under the chin. This helps relax the jaw and massages the lymph nodes in this area. After these facial strokes, turn your baby over on her tummy for the back massage.

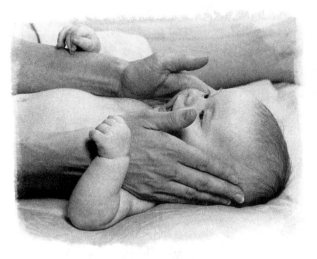

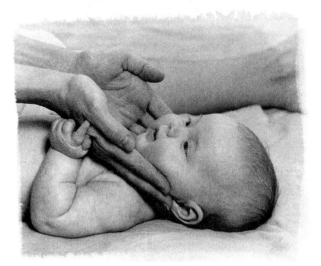

"May I Massage Your Back?"

The back is often a favorite with babies and toddlers alike. It can be the most relaxing part of the massage. These strokes also act as a warm-up for the gentle exercises that follow. To massage the back, turn your baby onto his tummy, either on the surface or on your lap with your legs extended. Older babies might like a toy to play with or a safe mirror to look at while the back is massaged.

1. RESTING HANDS

Position your baby and begin by relaxing yourself and letting the baby know the back massage is about to begin.

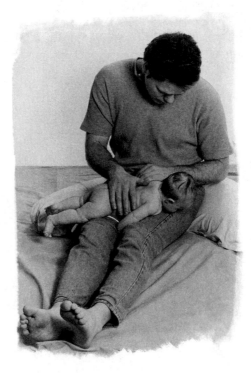

2. BACK AND FORTH

Start with both hands together at the top of the back, at right angles to the spine. Stroke your hands back and forth, perpendicular to the spine, alternating, molding your hands to the baby's back. Move down to the buttocks, then back up to the shoulders, then back down once again.

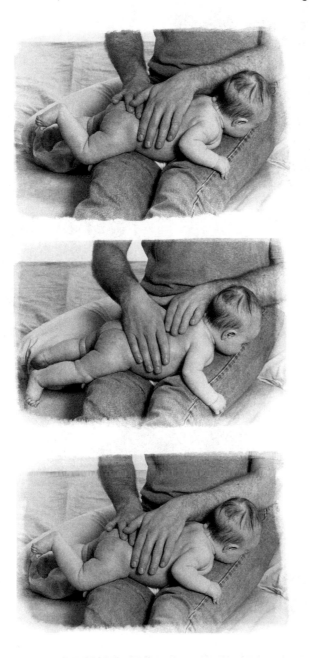

3. SWOOPING PART A

Keep one hand stationary under the bottom. Beginning at the shoulders, the other hand swoops down to meet the hand at the bottom. Mold your hand to the baby's back. Repeat several times.

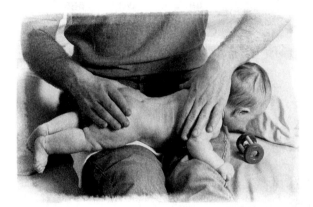

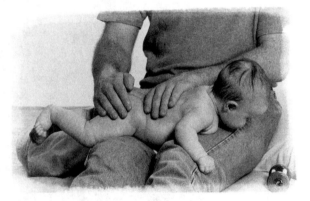

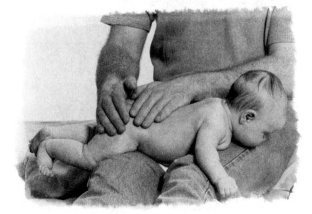

4. SWOOPING PART B

Holding one hand at your baby's feet (you may have to gently hold the feet still), swoop the other hand all the way down the back and the legs, to the ankles. Repeat several times.

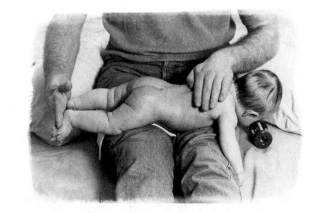

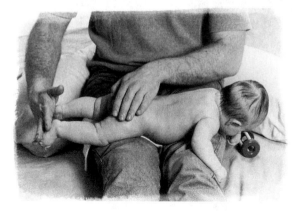

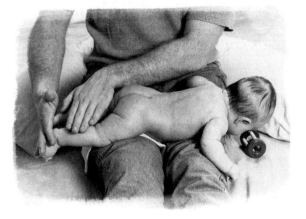

5. BACK CIRCLES

Make small circles all around the back with your fingertips. As your baby grows, you can feel muscles develop right under your fingertips!

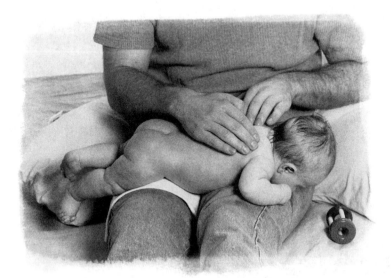

6. COMBING

To finish the back, make "combing" strokes from the shoulders to the lower back, with your fingers spread apart, each stroke getting lighter and lighter, ending with a "feather touch." This tells your baby you are finished with the back.

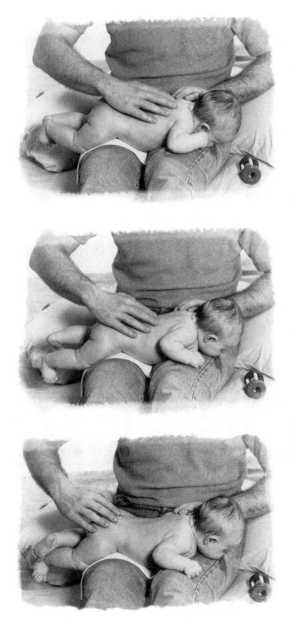

Gentle Movements

These movements are simple exercises that gently stretch baby's arms and legs, massage her stomach and pelvis, and align her spine. They are like yoga poses adapted for a baby. Be very gentle, and have fun with this routine, incorporating rhymes and games (see Chapter 18). After your baby begins to walk, these exercises will be unnecessary, as she will get plenty of stretching and exercise in day-to-day life.

1. CROSS ARMS

Cross your baby's arms at the chest three times, alternating which arm is over and under. Then gently stretch the arms out to the sides. The rhythm is: cross-cross-cross-open. Repeat.

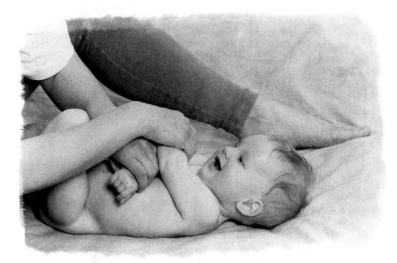

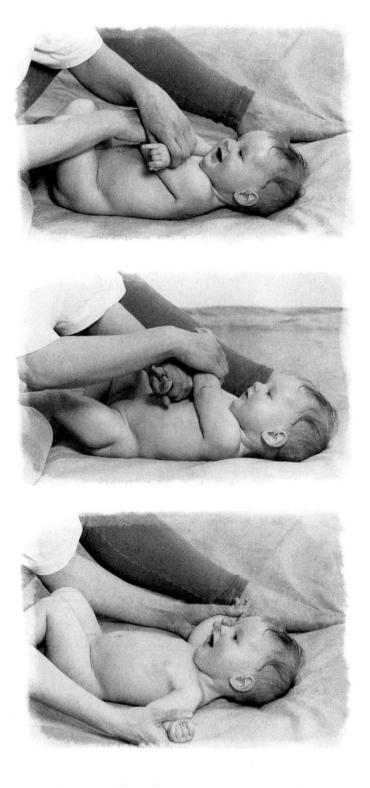

2. CROSS ARM AND LEG

Hold one arm at the wrist and the opposite leg at the ankle. Gently bring the arm down diagonally to the rib cage and the foot up diagonally toward the shoulder (allowing the knee to bend), then cross the leg and arm so that the arm goes to the outside of the leg, and cross again so the arm is under the leg, then cross once more with the arm over the leg. Now stretch them out in opposite directions. The rhythm is: cross-cross-cross-open. Repeat with the other arm and leg. Note: With an older baby, bring the knee, rather than the foot, up to cross with the arm.

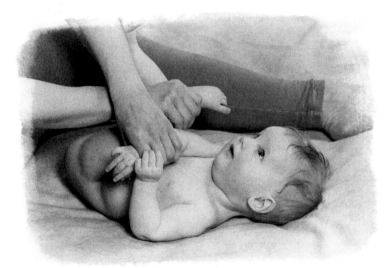

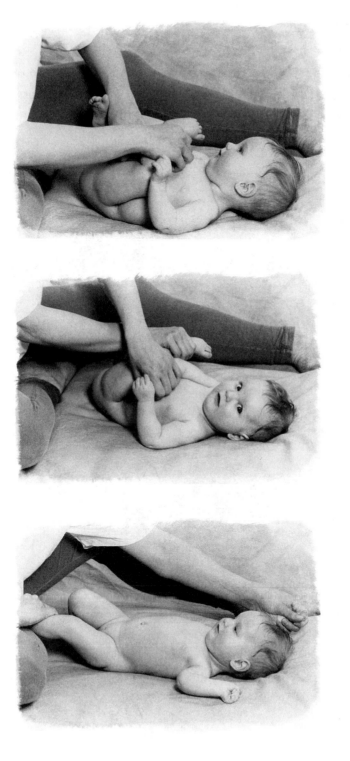

3. CROSS LEGS

Cross the legs over the tummy three times, alternating which leg is over and under. Then gently stretch the legs out straight, toward you, gently shaking and bouncing the legs to help relax. The rhythm is: cross-cross-cross-straighten. Repeat.

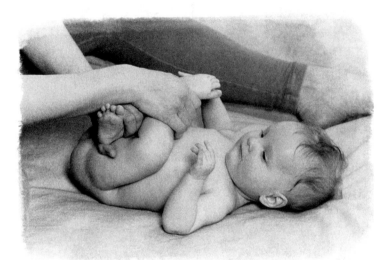

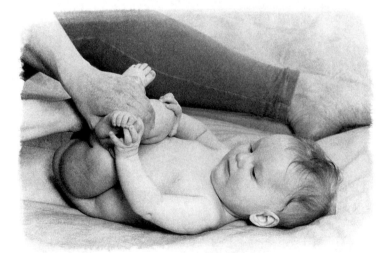

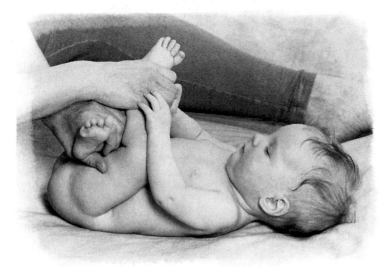

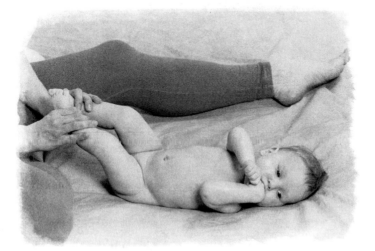

4. UP DOWN

Push the knees together up into the tummy, then stretch them out straight. If the baby resists straightening his legs, bounce them gently and encourage him to relax. Repeat several times.

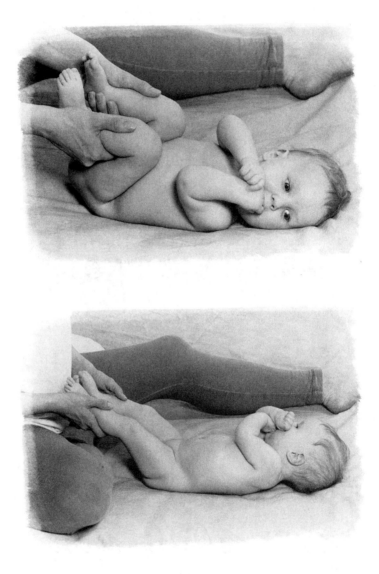

5. BICYCLE

Gently push the knees into the tummy, one after the other, then bounce them out straight to relax. The rhythm is push right—push left—push right—straighten, alternating the leg you start with each time.

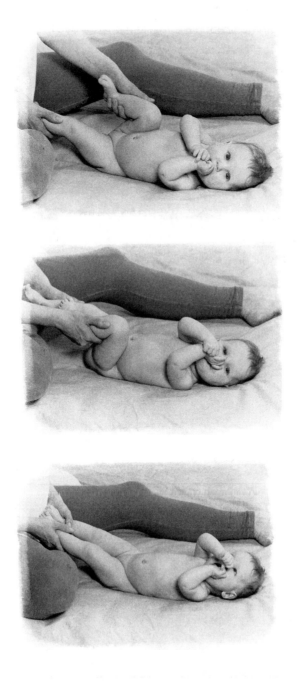

Abbreviated Massage

Sometimes you want to give your baby a quick massage on the run, when changing his diaper or just before bed. Here is an abbreviated massage that will take only a few minutes but will still provide the benefits of communication and relaxation your baby needs. This massage can be done with oil or lotion.

1. Rolling, on legs
2. Thumb Press, on soles of feet
3. Water Wheel Part A
4. Sun Moon and/or I Love You on tummy
5. Open Book, on chest
6. Rolling, on arms
7. Open Hand (with thumbs)
8. Finger Roll
9. Open Book, on forehead
10. Relax the Jaw
11. Back and Forth, on back
12. Combing, on back

Review of the Strokes

1. Relax and breathe deeply as you remove your jewelry and your baby's clothing, covering the genitals with a cloth or diaper.
2. Oil your palms and rub them together to warm them up.
3. Show your palms to your baby and request permission to begin.
4. Legs and feet:
     a. Resting Hands
     b. Indian Milking
     c. Hug and Glide
     d. Thumb over Thumb
     e. Toe Roll
     f. Under Toes
     g. Heel of Foot
     h. Thumb Press
     i. Top of Foot
     j. Ankle Circles
     k. Swedish Milking
     l. Rolling
     m. Bottom Relaxer
     n. Integration
     (Repeat with other leg)
5. Stomach:
     a. Resting Hands
     b. Water Wheel Part A and Part B
     c. Thumbs to Sides
     d. Sun Moon
     e. I Love You
     f. Walking
6. Chest:
     a. Resting Hands
     b. Open Book
     c. Butterfly
     d. Integration

7. Arms and Hands:

    a. Resting Hands

    b. Pit Stop

    c. Indian Milking

    d. Hug and Glide

    e. Finger Roll

    f. Top of Hand

    g. Wrist Circles

    h. Swedish Milking

    i. Rolling

    j. Touch Relaxation

    k. Integration

    (Repeat with other arm)

8. Face:

    a. Open Book

    b. Relax Your Eyes

    c. Happy Sinuses and Cheek Muscles

    d. Smile

    e. Relax the Jaw

    f. Ears, Neck, and All of Those Chins!

9. Back:

    a. Resting Hands

    b. Back and Forth

    c. Swooping Part A and Part B

    d. Back Circles

    e. Combing

10. Gentle Movements:

    a. Cross Arms

    b. Cross Arm and Leg

    c. Cross Legs

    d. Up Down

    e. Bicycle

11. And a kiss to grow on!

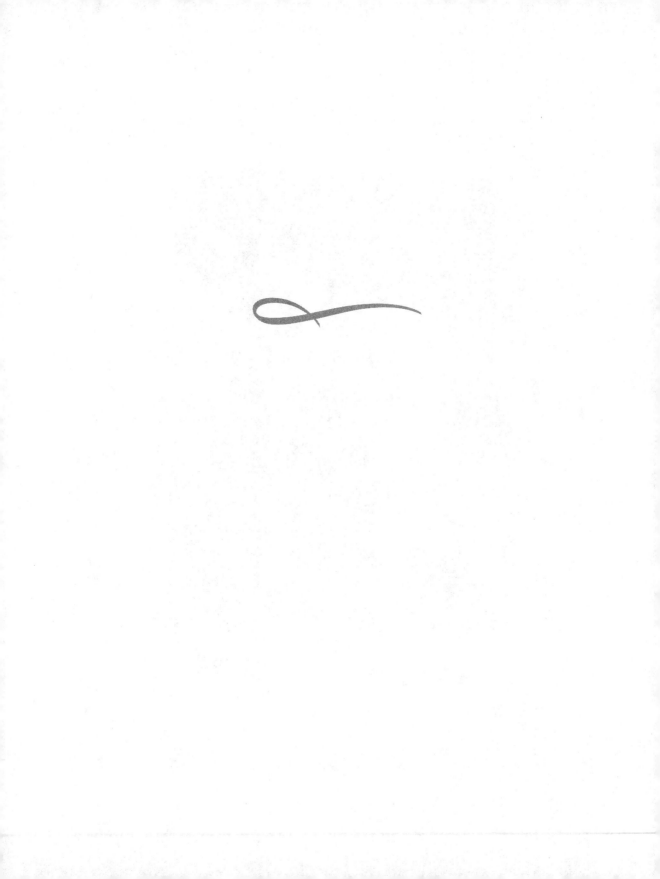

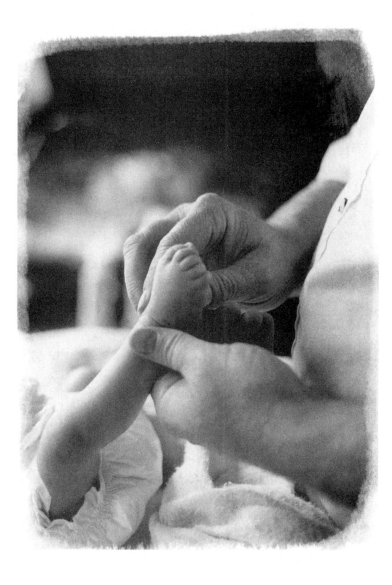

Chapter 14

Crying, Fussing, and Other Baby Language (Including Cues, Reflexes, and Behavioral States)

This is my sad time of day.

—ARNOLD LOBEL,

FROG AND TOAD ARE FRIENDS

Babies Fuss and Cry—That's What They Do!

At this point, you may be imagining yourself lovingly massaging your baby as he lies there contentedly listening to your voice, gazing into your eyes, and perhaps even falling asleep. This will probably happen quite often, and when it does, it is wonderful. But most babies will fuss or cry at times during a massage. If you understand the reasons for your baby's fussiness, you will be much more comfortable and better able to help him.

Because infants grow so rapidly, there is often much tension in their little bodies. They work so hard to develop muscle coordination that occasionally they may well ache and feel out of sorts.

When your body aches, a massage feels both good and uncomfortable at the same time. Your muscles are sore, and even a gentle touch can bring discomfort. Still, being touched is so relaxing, and getting blood circulating through your sore muscles is so healing, that your grunts and grimaces may mean both pain and pleasure. Often a massage can remind you of aches you never knew you had, but afterward the feelings of relief and release you experience are well worth it.

Massage is a new experience for your little one. At first she may react negatively to the sensations she experiences, as they are so new, but after she becomes accustomed to being touched in this fashion, she will begin to enjoy the routine. So take it easy at first, and acquaint her with these new sensations slowly. You, too, may feel clumsy and flustered at first, trying to learn the strokes and do them "correctly," leading to tension on your part, which your baby will pick up.

Babies who had a difficult or traumatic birth, who had difficulties afterward for which they needed medical intervention, or who have just come from foster homes or orphanages tend to have more negative reactions to being massaged at first. For example, babies who have received routine heel sticks for blood testing often cry when their feet are massaged, even several months later. If your baby seems to be reacting negatively to particular parts of the massage, use Touch Relaxation techniques and gentle Resting Hands first, gradually introducing massage strokes as they are accepted.

Fussing

Some babies need time to become accustomed to being massaged and will, at first, become fussy after just a few minutes. Breathe deeply, and make every effort to relax yourself. Then allow the baby to fuss a little. Often he will release the tension during the massage, and the massage itself will make him a lot happier, more relaxed, and able to sleep more soundly. As tension is released and the baby's stimulation threshold rises, the fussing will diminish.

If your baby consistently begins to fuss at a certain point in the massage, it may be that he needs a break, or a shorter massage period for a while. You can take a break to nurse or cuddle, then try again. If he continues to fuss, you may try massaging for a shorter period, at a different time of day, or starting on a different area of the body. Check to be sure he is warm enough, that you are relaxed and comfortable, and that there is no outside stimulation such as radio, television, computer, or phone. Listen closely to what he says with his fussing; perhaps he needs to tell you about his day! Check for gas or colic, and listen, listen, listen. Your baby has a lot to say and needs to be heard.

When Your Baby Is "Disorganized"

Sometimes your baby will fuss and cry because he feels overstimulated, in pain, stressed out, tired, and unable to gather his energies back together and either rest or go to sleep. Mothers worldwide have invented many techniques to help babies when they feel "disorganized." Holding her in the manner she likes while rocking or walking her can help. Sometimes a warm bath can help. Some parents even drive the baby around in the car!

Dr. Robert Hamilton of Pacific Ocean Pediatrics in Santa Monica, California, invented a marvelous way to soothe out-of-sorts, crying babies (particularly in the first three months). In an interview with ABC News, Hamilton said, "Typically, when you examine children, they cry. That's what we expect as pediatricians. What I found over time is that after I gave them a shot, clearly they started to cry and I thought, 'Okay, I broke it, I have to fix it.'" So as he spoke to the parents, he had a little method that evolved over the years. He would gently lift the baby up and down, and wrap the baby's arms across the chest with his left hand. "That was the element that comforted them more than anything," he says. The baby would calm down, and the parents would ask how to do it themselves.

"I very gently wrap the two arms right in front of the chest, I put him in a prone position," Hamilton said as he demonstrated live on *Good Morning America*. "Then with my dominant hand, I grab his little bottom and very gently rock him up and down. Sometimes they'll grab your finger and suck on it. It works very, very well." The doctor's instructional video was an Internet sensation, racking up more than fifteen million views. "Remember where they came from," said Hamilton. "They came from very, very tight quarters, if you will. And by folding the arms you're essentially swaddling them. They recognize that position."

Hamilton says he's been doing this for about twenty years. "All of this is very gentle," he says. He sometimes refers to it as "shaking their booty." It's not a surprise that his mentor and friend is Harvey Karp, the pediatrician who made the "shhhh" method famous in the book *The Happiest Baby on the Block*.

The technique I saw done most often in India was one I found to be useful with my babies and many of the babies in my classes. I call it Indian Bouncing, and it is very simple. You lay your baby across your lap, facedown, making sure he has room to breathe, parting your legs a bit for his tummy. Be sure your baby's head is supported to prevent harming his delicate neck; let the baby's cheek or chin rest on a folded blanket or towel on your legs. Never let baby's head hang off your leg. Then lay warm, relaxed Resting Hands on his back. Now, very gently bounce your knees up and down rhythmically and slowly, as you gently pat your baby's back at the same rate with slightly cupped hands.

Do this rhythmic bouncing for about five minutes. Usually the baby will either fall asleep or stop fussing and relax into the rhythm. If and when he feels centered again, you may put him down for a nap or carry on with your day. When I traveled by train in India, I often observed mothers in groups with their babies across their knees, patting and bouncing them as they talked to one another. Everyone seemed to be having a wonderful time! In the orphanage where I worked and in Mother Teresa's baby hospital, this method was also used, with swaddling, to help a baby or toddler whose energies seemed out of control.

Why Babies Cry

Babies cry for many reasons, and it is important to learn your baby's personality and his different cries so that you can respond to them. There are cries that mean "I need affection," "I'm hungry," "I'm in pain," or "I'm tired and cranky and don't know how to get to sleep," and still others that are simply "venting" for all the stress the baby takes in as she adjusts to the world of nonstop stimulation. Each of these different cries can and should be responded to specifically. Each baby will differ in his or her need for physical affection. Some need to be held nearly all the time for the first few months; others are curious and independent almost immediately. To force an infant one way or another is to disempower her and disrupt the flow of *chi* (vital energy) she needs to become strong, healthy, and independent.

There has been at least one app invented to tell parents why their baby is crying. Don't fall for these claims—they are intended to make a quick profit from desperate parents, and in my experience they do not work. The way to respond to your baby is to listen, listen, listen, and use your intuition and experience to guide your responses.

Some folks think that babies who cry always need to be calmed and shushed, or, conversely, should be left alone to cry it out. This is not true. Infants should never be left alone to cry, unheeded, but sometimes they need to cry in the safety of a parent's arms, without being shushed, to discharge stress. After a certain period, when they sense they are being attended to, they calm and usually sleep much more deeply.

According to the latest research, women who experience stress, worry, or panic attacks before and/or during pregnancy are more than twice as likely to report that their babies cried "excessively." Researchers reported that mothers suffering from anxiety may have a more "intrusive" parenting style that could cause babies to cry more.

Experts suggest an infant's excessive crying may be due to the mother's production of stress hormones during pregnancy, which may cross the placenta and affect the development of a baby's brain. In an article from

Dailymail.com titled "Mothers who experience stress or worry before pregnancy 'more likely to have babies who cry for longer'," by Jo MacFar-lane, a parenting specialist, Dr. Clare Bailey, says, "Mothers can easily get into a traumatic negative cycle when worrying about a newborn child. The more they worry, the less they sleep and calm themselves down and the more they worry. Anxiety can make them hypervigilant, distressed by crying, and even rejected by their child. It intuitively sounds likely that a calm mother feeling relaxed, comfortable and confident will be more likely to help a child regulate its crying, while an anxious mother may be less likely to help a baby to self-settle. Babies can pick up emotional cues very early on."

It is possible for stress hormones to cross the placenta and contribute to an infant's crying spells. Infant massage addresses this by (1) helping the baby's gastrointestinal system mature, (2) addressing the baby's (and parent's) need for close, loving contact, and (3) helping parents feel empowered to help their infants feel secure, loved, and bonded to their parents.

This is one of the important reasons to massage your pregnant belly and to massage your infant regularly after birth. You learn, as nothing else can teach you, what your baby needs, and her cries and fusses don't distress you so much as inform you of what you need to do to respond appropriately and thus allow your child to grow and blossom like a well-tended flower in your garden. If you respond in these ways, you needn't worry about when to wean, when to potty-train, and all the other advice people want to give you. You will become an expert on your child, and you will naturally know and understand what she is ready to do and when. This gives you the confidence to listen to the so-called experts and then go by your inner sense of what is right.

"Cry It Out"

One modern parenting practice that has attracted a rethink by experts is that of the belief that leaving babies to "cry it out" for periods of time is good for them. These practices might have made sense to some, but science has now discovered that they are not at all helpful to an infant.

In the 1880s behavioral psychologist John Watson believed that emotional distance-keeping was the key to raising independent children. The latest in medical advice at the time was to put babies down without rocking or nursing them to sleep, and not to respond to their cries. A great concern about germs and infection caused medical professionals to campaign against affection—warning mothers about the risk of too much touching. According to Watson, who was president of the American Psychological Association, if mothers were too kind to their infants, they would end up with a dependent, demanding child who leads his parents around by the nose. There was no evidence to back up these claims, but rather proof everywhere (both then and now) that touching, love, and affection meet the babies' needs and help them grow up to be happy, independent human beings with strong bonds with their parents and the ability to create strong, healthy bonds with others (including their own children).

The attitude that too much contact between mothers and their infants was a waste of time and that the baby should never, ever inconvenience mom are well-known to us today. Many of our parents and grandparents repeated these ideas to their kids having babies. Now, neuroscience tells us that allowing infants to suffer anguish and despair can damage them and their ability to properly relate to others in the long term. The child learns that she must scream, and even then, she cannot expect attention to her needs. Leaving infants to "cry it out" creates more fearful, uncooperative, alienated people who will pass the same or worse habits to the following generation. Such children learn not to ask for help and attention, and potentially withdraw into depression and their health is compromised.

According to Darcia Narvaez, Ph.D., in an article for *Psychology Today*, "Instead, giving babies what they need leads to greater independence later. In anthropological reports of small-band hunter-gatherers, parents take care of every need of babies and young children." She goes on, "Babies indicate a need through gesture and eventually, if necessary, through crying. Just as adults reach for liquid when they are thirsty, children search for what they need in the moment. Just as adults become calm once the need is met, so do babies."

How "Cry It Out" Affects Babies

A baby's brain is damaged in several ways. The interconnections between nerve cells is impaired; anguish creates the conditions for the destruction of synapses (junctions between nerve cells), which contribute to the connectivity and efficiency of the networks being built in the brain. Early brain development is the foundation of human adaptability and resilience (the capacity to recover quickly from difficulties). During this period of distress, the hormone cortisol is released, which can cause several cascading effects, including:

- inadequately functioning vagus nerve, related to disorders such as irritable bowel syndrome
- shutting down when experiencing substantial distress—stop growing, feeling, trusting
- the development of mistrust in relationships; the undermining of self-confidence, resulting in an inner emptiness that a child may take a lifetime trying to fill

Notre Dame professor of psychology Darcia Narvaez, Ph.D. says, "Responsiveness to crying, almost constant touch and having multiple adult caregivers are some of the nurturing ancestral parenting practices that are shown to positively impact the developing brain, which not only shapes personality, but also helps physical health and moral development."

A parent is also affected by ignoring an infant's crying. He learns to ignore more subtle cues about the baby's needs. The relationship between parent and infant is broken by the parent, but can't be repaired by the child; the infant is powerless.

Research from NYU Langone Medical Center found that a mother's presence soothes pain for a crying baby and it also can influence brain development by altering gene activity in the part of the brain involved in emotions. According to neurobiologist Regina Sullivan, Ph.D., "Our study shows that a mother comforting her infant in pain does not just elect a behavioral response, but also the comforting modifies—for better or worse—critical neural circuitry during early brain development."

What Is It About Crying Anyway?

Once I was asked to demonstrate infant massage for a television news spot. As we hurried to the newsroom, the host said, "I hear you have a way to stop a baby's screams in ten seconds flat with massage. I hope you can show us that today!"

The baby, a sweet four-month-old with whom I'd had a lovely conversation in the greenroom, took one look at the newscaster and began to cry inconsolably. I did not demonstrate massage because I felt it would betray her feelings to use it as a trick to quiet her (even if it could have, which I doubt). The host concluded that the infant massage gimmick did not work. She was right—as a gimmick, it does not. Unfortunately, this was not the only time I was confronted with this "quick fix" mentality. Many people still think that babies should be seen and not heard.

Why do babies cry so much? Why does it bother adults so much? Why are people so confused about how to respond to a crying infant? As infants, we had few ways beyond crying to express negative feelings and release pent-up stress. While growing up, we learned how to deal with anger, fear, pain, and excess energy in many ways; our facial expressions, body language, and speech patterns now help us to convey how we feel. When the stresses of living pile up, we can go for a walk, take a vacation, or talk to a friend. Even when we are healthy, we cry from time to time. But we rarely cry in front of others.

We have learned that crying is antisocial and a sign of weakness. This was probably one of our earliest lessons.

Do Babies Manipulate Parents with Crying?

The injunction not to "spoil" a baby came into vogue in the early part of this century. People began to think that they should let babies "cry it out" alone. The rationale was that babies used crying to manipulate parents into gratifying their desires, and that this was an unattractive character trait. Responding to it could only cultivate spoiled, boorish children leading their parents around by the nose. In order to teach babies that crying was unacceptable behavior and to train them for independence early on, they were left alone to cry until they grew hoarse and fell asleep from sheer exhaustion.

In the 1970s, a movement away from these earlier infant-rearing practices gained momentum. Many more women began breastfeeding, the front and back packs were invented, and even baby experts such as Dr. T. Berry Brazelton recanted earlier advice not to take a baby into the parents' bed. We finally realized that, like fruit, the only way to spoil a baby is through neglect. Other cultures influenced this change; global communication had become sophisticated enough for us to begin looking more closely at cultures on the other side of the world that had not yet been impaired by so-called modern thinking.

Unfortunately, most Western cultures already had. Mothers who previously might have left their baby alone to cry while they felt guilty and tearful in the other room now jumped at the baby's smallest peep. But something still remained of that earlier mind-set. Getting the baby to stop crying, or not allowing the baby to cry at all, was still our obsession.

Today, in many people's minds, the pendulum has swung back to the thinking that babies become spoiled by being attended to and that they should be trained or "managed" to act according to what is convenient for their parents. It seems that regardless of where we are on this continuum, we continually miss the point regarding a baby's need to cry.

At times we all need to cry. It is a release, and crying in the loving arms of another is often much more so. I believe that babies' feelings are as deep as ours, that their fears, their sorrows, and their frustrations are not less. From observing hundreds of babies in massage classes and in other cultures, I know that sometimes crying can be a relief and release for them, and that often after a good cry they are happier, their digestion improves, and they sleep more deeply. This "good cry," however, can occur only in a loving, supportive atmosphere, where the baby is neither ignored nor hushed. The parent recognizes a cry of hunger or physical pain, or a need for cuddling, and responds appropriately to it.

Many of us brought up in the age of "don't spoil the baby" have mixed feelings about crying. We get anxious, tense up, and want the crying to stop right away. It triggers fear and perhaps a reminder of the anguish (and anger) we may have felt, crying alone in a crib with no response. It can also engender guilt—am I a bad mother if my baby cries?

Our culture reinforces these feelings. Many people are extremely agitated by any noise a baby makes and assail its parent with dour looks at the slightest sound. The embarrassed parent often responds by punishing the baby with loud hisses, apologizing for the baby, and fleeing for the safety of home. It does little good to recoil in shock at the statistics on battered children when our entire cultural setup actually creates this behavior. Battering is an extreme example, but almost all of us are caught in this cycle in one way or another. Most new parents in our culture periodically experience high levels of stress, regardless of their philosophies. Who has not had thoughts of "throwing the baby out the window" or fears of losing control and shaking or screaming at a crying baby?

When you are overwhelmed by these feelings, if possible ask your partner to hold the baby while you remove yourself to a quiet place for five or ten minutes to practice Controlled Belly Breathing and release your anxiety. If you feel so frustrated that you want to cry, go ahead. When my children were babies, we sometimes paced the living room together, both mother and baby crying through our pain and frustration. We should begin to accept crying as simply another way we humans can cleanse our hearts of negative feelings and stress. We can acknowledge that it is okay to cry sometimes, and that everyone eventually stops crying and finds relief, especially if their family and friends allow them to express their feelings, and love and respect them all the more for doing so.

Researchers have discovered that we have a built-in, instinctual response to an infant's cries. In several experiments, one-day-old infants became distressed upon hearing another infant's cries, but not upon hearing a synthesized, fake cry or the cry of an older child.

This suggests that the "distress response" is innate. How we act upon this distress, however, is determined by cultural factors. Western culture, as it has developed over the last hundreds of years, has systematically reduced our sensitivity to infants' cues and placed an unnatural distance between parents and babies and between family and community members. This split between "nature" and "nurture" has created a vicious cycle of crying babies, sleepless nights, and sometimes abuse.

Brazelton's and Mead's observations and studies of several nonindustrialized cultures show virtually continuous contact between mother and baby. Cultural patterns characterized by close mother-infant contact and prolonged breastfeeding also foster a highly developed sensitivity to baby signals and subtle cues, such as body movements and facial expressions that precede crying. This does not mean, however, that babies in these cultures never cry. While they rarely cry during the day, it is quite common for infants to cry for long periods in the evening. Adults know this is release crying and allow it. As Sandy Jones says in *Crying Babies, Sleepless Nights,* "There's a difference between not responding, and responding and allowing, in which you've used your judgment about what your baby seems to need." People in these cultures, because of their own experience of responsive parenting and a strong social support system, are quite able to automatically and naturally discriminate between a baby's distressed crying out for help and other kinds of communication. The baby's cry rarely pushes the parent into egoistic impulses.

Researchers have found that people respond to babies' cries in either an egoistic or an altruistic manner. Egoistic responses are characterized by agitation and concern with self; one wants to stop the baby's crying because it is aggravating. Altruistic responses are characterized by empathic discomfort; one wants to alleviate the baby's suffering. Egoism and altruism are fostered by both biology and culture. Maternal hormones, such as prolactin, have been shown to be a factor in an altruistic response to infant crying; these hormones are elevated by extended contact and breastfeeding. Our culture in many ways encourages and cultivates egoism. We have isolated people more and more over the last several generations. Thus, the social support network for most new parents is often nonexistent. The demands of our economy and our social values motivate both parents to provide financial income, often at the cost of increased stress for parents and infants.

Studies reveal that the social support network is very closely related to the security of the parent-infant bond. A lack of external support can distance parents from their babies and thus threaten the baby's healthy development. Babies who are "high-need"—colicky, hypersensitive criers—are especially vulnerable to abuse and neglect in situations where parents are suffering marital or financial difficulties. A good social support system can mitigate problems between baby and parent. Unresponsive mothers who are given a lot of support, help, encouragement, and physical affection can become responsive to their babies, and babies who have a lot of contact with loving friends, grandparents, and caregivers are not as affected by difficulties in the mother-infant attachment. The philosophies of the behaviorists spawned several generations of people who lacked the basic security of a strong parental bond. We, and many of our parents and grandparents, grew up concerned with our own security above all; the anxious attachment created by the anti-spoiling atmosphere of infancy could only bring about self-concern.

The result of this culturally promoted egoism is an overall lack of responsiveness to babies, which fosters more crying. Silvia Bell and Mary Ainsworth's studies showed that not responding properly to babies' cries in the first six months actually increases the frequency of crying and distress in the next six months and later. Violence is an egoistic response. According to B. F. Steele and C. B. Pollock's work, abusive parents (often the victims of abuse themselves) frequently have extreme views about spoiling and independence training—views handed down and culturally reinforced—that contribute to their baby's distress, thus further agitating the already stressed parent. In addition, these views inhibit close contact, carrying, and breastfeeding, thus lowering the chances of hormonal support for sympathetic responses.

Like all of us, babies have many different reasons for crying. Unfortunately, we have lost much of our capacity to intuit their thoughts and feelings. Most people are able to recognize a sharp cry of pain, but our interpretations of other cries and fusses are filtered through the veil of our own insecurities and projections. It may be easier to adopt a mechanistic philosophy, whereby one always responds in the same way, either ignoring or hushing. But babies are not interested in philosophy and are unable to attend to their parent's (or anyone else's) comfort. To begin to get a more centered awareness, observe yourself when your baby (or someone else's) cries. When you understand your reactions, you will be able to begin to understand the baby. Notice what a crying baby stimulates for you. Breathe deeply, relax your body, and perhaps think of an affirmation such as "I release fear and tension, and go with love to comfort my baby."

Dr. William Sears, author of *The Fussy Baby*, advises parents to picture several response buttons on their "internal computer." "If your baby cries and you push the right response button," he says, "there is an inner feeling of rightness about your response." Daily massage can be an aid in this process, because it helps you to literally keep in touch with your baby's body language and nonverbal signals. Changing our society begins at home. Even so, there are opportunities to influence the culture beyond our own doorstep. We can help grandparents, friends, and prospective parents gain awareness of babies' needs. We can make an effort to provide support and encouragement to friends with new infants. We can also model consideration of babies at social functions and in public.

Actively and compassionately listening to an infant isn't much different from listening to a child or adult. It requires empathy, genuine love, and respect for the person's experience. The reason it is so difficult for us to listen to our babies, I believe, is that our own infancies may have been full of frustration and unheard feelings. When we hear our babies cry, rather than truly listening to what they are saying, we superimpose our own "inner infant." Our overwhelming impulse is to quiet that baby. We hush our babies as we ourselves were hushed.

Research has consistently shown that babies who are responded to promptly—not by hushing but by listening and acting—cry less frequently and for shorter periods as they grow older. Crying releases hormones that reduce tension and arousal. It is not only an expression of pain or discomfort but seems to be an inborn stress-management and healing mechanism. If allowed and responded to with relaxed, loving listening, crying can help babies regulate their own stress levels and grow to be more relaxed and stress-free children and adults.

How to Listen to a Baby

When your baby begins to vocalize, fuss, or cry during massage, you can use a three-step process. First, take a long, slow, deep breath and relax your whole body. This directly counteracts the tendency to hold your breath and tighten up. Tell yourself, "No big deal."

Second, set aside your own inner infant for a moment. In order to truly hear your baby, you must clear yourself and realize that your baby has his own reasons for crying. Third, make eye contact with your baby if possible. If he is avoiding eye contact, place your hands gently but firmly on his body, and connect with him through your hands. Let your love go to him, telling him with your voice, your eyes, and your hands that you would like to hear what he has to say.

Stay with the baby, keeping yourself very relaxed and receptive. Listen and respond to him, observing his body language. Watch his mouth and what he says with his eyes. When you are sure he feels heard and has said most of what he has to say, offer the comfort of rocking, walking, bouncing, and cuddling to help him get organized again. Invariably, a baby who feels he has been heard will sleep more deeply afterward and will extend himself in trust more the next time.

When we truly listen to our infants, we are fulfilling all of their psychological needs. Our underlying message is, "You are worthy of respect. You are valuable just the way you are." The baby takes in this message, and her whole body relaxes. The chalice of her heart is filled to overflowing, and as she grows, she will seek opportunities to share her love with others. How will she do this? By following the model she has been given. She will be there for others in the way you have been there for her. What a lovely, healthy cycle!

Your Baby's Cues

Your baby has a lot to say but has not yet developed language. So he uses his body language, facial expressions, cries, coos, and other sounds to communicate with you. Pay close attention to these signals. Your baby is teaching you his unique way of saying what he wants you to hear. Dr. Linda Acredolo and Dr. Susan Goodwyn, authors of *Baby Signs: How to Talk with Your Baby Before Your Baby Can Talk,* recognized this tendency in babies to "sign" before learning speech. In their fascinating book, they show how babies make up signs for objects and feelings and teach them to their parents. The parents, if they are conscious of them, can then use the signs with their babies and attach words to them, so when a baby is ready to speak, the word comes easily. Later on, parents can also teach their babies signs for things, showing a sign and attaching a word to it, to help the baby develop language before speech. For example, a one-year-old may open and close her hands to indicate "book."

This way of "talking" before speech can be important to us in our babies' massage routine. Your palms swishing together can come to mean "massage," and asking your baby's permission further indicates that a massage is being offered. Often when a baby is feeling stressed out by the stimulation, she will give a sign or cue to let you know she needs a break. She may, for example, hold a hand up in front of her face as if to say, "Stop!" Sometimes hiccuping is a stress cue. If she looks around rapidly while fussing, she may need to be swaddled and comforted and/or rhythmically rocked or bounced to bring her energies back into alignment and calm her.

I encourage you to begin teaching your baby signs for "massage," "no," and "relax" (perhaps wiggling limp hands while saying the word "relax"), signs for the various body parts, signs for "happy," "sad," and "angry," and a sign for "all done," even before the baby is capable of giving the signs back to you. Acredolo and Goodwyn say that baby signs will usually not be used until a baby is about nine months old. But other researchers have found that even in the premature nursery, babies give "cues" to alert their caregivers of their state and their needs. You will learn your own baby's unique cues as you massage him day by day. Not all babies mean the same thing when they hiccup, hold up a hand, or look away. Allow your baby to teach you what he means by the various signs he gives you through his body language. Often during a massage, a baby will go through a very short period of stress-release fussing, in which he gives these stress cues, but then settles down and enjoys the rest of the massage. The idea is simply to be aware of your baby's unique expressions and to help her give words to her gestures so that when she is ready to talk, she knows exactly what to say.

Your Newborn's Reflexes

During massage, you may notice that your newborn has some automatic responses to different kinds of stimulation. These are called reflexes. Observe your newborn carefully, and you will see these reflexes happen. Nothing to be concerned about!

Rooting
When massaging your newborn's face, she may respond with the rooting reflex: turning her head to the side. This may happen as you stroke past the

edge of the mouth when doing the upper lip and lower lip Smile strokes. You may also notice this reflex when doing the Relax the Jaw strokes.

Startle (Moro)

When a newborn experiences a loud noise or sudden change in position or when his head drops backward, the baby will extend his arms and legs and then pull them back quickly. As you lay your baby on the floor in front of you, you may notice a startle response. If there is a sudden movement or loud noise, you may also notice this reflex.

Plantar/Grasping

When you touch the sole of your newborn's foot, her toes curl down toward the sole of the foot.

Palmar/Grasping

When you stroke the palm or put your finger in your newborn's palm, he will grab on tightly. Babies from their first days to six months of age instinctively grasp objects placed in their palm and are able to distinguish among different objects by feel. The grasping response is called the palmar reflex. It fades when your baby is around six months due to his more sophisticated motor skills, which allow him to consciously grasp objects for himself. Babies will often explore by oral touch, grabbing objects and putting them into their mouths to feel them.

Asymmetrical Tonic Neck Reflex (ATNR)

During any part of the massage, the ATNR reflex may be stimulated. You may see your newborn's head turn to one side as she arches her body and extends an arm/leg out in a "fencing" position: arm/leg extended in the same direction as the infant's turned head is facing, other arm/leg flexed.

Babinski

When you stroke the outside of the sole of the foot or top of the foot, adjacent to the toes, the newborn's toes straighten out.

Babkin

When you press the palms of both hands simultaneously, your newborn's mouth opens and the head bends toward the chest. The hand may come to the mouth.

Your Baby's Behavioral States

It's good to know about your baby's behavioral states so that you can choose to massage him at the most beneficial time for both of you. Here are the basic states through which your baby moves throughout the day:

Quiet Alert: The Best State for Infant Massage
- Little to no body movement
- Eyes are wide open and bright
- Gazing at faces
- Responding to voices
- The state in which baby is most open to learning

Active Alert: Another Good Time for Infant Massage
- Frequent movement
- Eyes scan, searching for people and objects
- Small vocalizations (coos, gurgles, grunts)

Crying
- Physical: hungry, soiled diapers, too hot/cold, tired, in pain
- Emotional: lonely, scared, over- or understimulated, bored

Drowsy
- Occurs while baby is waking up or falling asleep
- Eyes have a dull, glazed appearance and do not focus
- Eyelids are droopy

Quiet Sleep

- Relaxed face
- Still eyes and lids
- Still body, occasional startles
- Slow and even breathing
- Deep sighs every so often

Active Sleep

- Varied facial expressions (smiles, frowns, sucking)
- REM sleep—rapid eye movement under the lids
- Occasional body movement
- Irregular breathing
- Vocalizations (squeaks, grunts, gurgles)

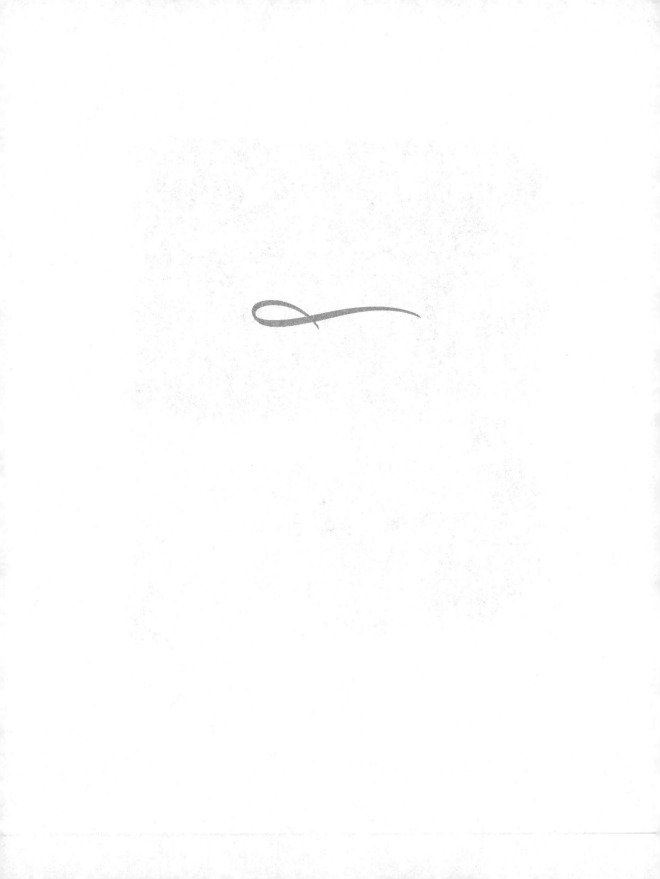

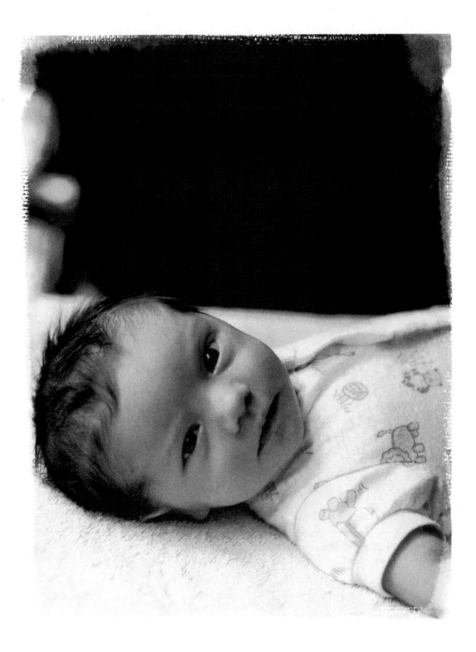

Chapter 15

Minor Illness and Colic

Can a mother sit and hear
An infant groan, an infant fear?
No, no! never can it be!
Never, never can it be!

—WILLIAM BLAKE, "ON ANOTHER'S SORROW"

Some Simple Suggestions

In times of illness, a massage not only can comfort but also can help relieve painful symptoms such as aches, fever, congestion, and the labored breathing of croup and asthma. Of course, as with any significant deviation from health in your baby, consult your family doctor about its use.

Fever

To help bring down a fever, use some of the same strokes as in the basic massage. Use warm water on your hands instead of oil, and except for the part you are working on, keep the baby's body covered. Working from the chest to the extremities, dip your hand in the water, then briskly rub the body. The idea is to bring the heat up to the surface of the skin, where the water will evaporate and help cool it. Whenever the baby has a fever, check with the physician. My own baby's pediatrician taught me this method as a way to bring down a fever when my baby had ear infections.

Chest Congestion

You can use another technique to help ease chest congestion. First, do the regular massage strokes for the chest, using oil on your hands, adding a drop of eucalyptus oil or a dab of Mentholatum ointment. Tip the baby at a slight angle on your lap, with his head down. Using a small cup (the clean plastic cup from the top of a cough syrup bottle works nicely) or something with a small rim, press in and pull out gently all over his chest and back. The gentle suction helps pull mucus away from the lungs so it can be coughed up. A vaporizer in the baby's room can help, too. Be sure the vaporizer is very clean so it is not putting harmful bacteria into the air. This method is useful for baby croup and asthma as well. Again, consult with the baby's pediatrician first.

Nasal Congestion

For nasal congestion, assemble the following: a nasal aspirator, a dropper, a washcloth, and a cup of warm salted water (ratio: one-half teaspoon salt per cup of warm water). Do the massage strokes for the face, especially the ones for the sinus area, to help relax the area, increase circulation, and loosen mucus. Place a drop of the warm salted water in each nostril. Push the bulb end of the aspirator closed. Now, carefully and gently insert the aspirator tip into the baby's nostril. Release the pressure on the bulb and suction out the mucus with the aspirator, closing it into the washcloth. The warm salt water is easy on her nose and will help loosen the mucus considerably. She will not enjoy this process, but it may be necessary if her stuffiness is preventing her from sucking, and it is better to avoid using over-the-counter medicines if possible. Her own antibodies will fight the cold and will be stronger next time in immunizing her against viruses. After you are finished, comfort the baby and feed her. Be sure you clean all of the items very carefully with boiling water, to kill any micro-organisms, before using them again.

Gas and Colic

Babies often cry because of painful gas or because they are tired and their energies are disorganized. Discomfort and outright pain from trapped gas are very common. Since babies' gastrointestinal systems are immature at birth, they need prompting to begin functioning the way they should. Massage can provide just the right type of stimulation.

All babies cry, but some babies fuss and cry (even screech!) for hours every day. Many new parents quickly learn that for some babies, feeding, changing a diaper, adjusting the temperature, or cuddling doesn't make their infant stop wailing. Usually when an infant cries for hours at a time, seemingly in pain, pediatricians tell parents the baby has "colic," and they say, "Don't worry, it will go away after three or four months." Parents re-coil at this; tired and frustrated, they scour the Web and survey doctors and other parents, searching for something—anything—to end their ba-by's discomfort due to infantile colic.

I learned early on, from practice with my own baby and from others in my infant massage classes, that colic is caused by an underdeveloped gas-trointestinal system. I developed a Colic Relief Routine including massage strokes and yoga postures that, if done religiously every day, virtually eliminates colic within two weeks. My foundation for this practice is not a double-blind study but years of observation and working directly with parents of colicky babies. They are so relieved that they do not have to wait months for the crying to be finished!

"Infantile colic is one of the major concerns of many parents of ba-bies, and for a long time, doctors and parents alike have struggled with a lack of treatment options to ease colic symptoms in early infancy," says

Dr. Gideon Koren, director of the Motherisk Program and senior scientist at The Hospital for Sick Children in Toronto. An estimated 5 to 40 percent of infants experience colic, typically ending at about three or four months. Babies with colic usually cry, seemingly in pain, at least three hours a day, more than three days a week, over at least three weeks, with no obvious trigger. While recognized by the medical community for centuries, the cause of infantile colic remains unknown by the pediatric community, with theories ranging from overproduction of intestinal gas to insecure parental attachment. Some research has pointed to a potential role for intestinal microbiota, microorganisms that include "good bacteria," which differ greatly between infants with colic and those without. Some babies with colic have been shown to have inadequate levels of a type of good bacteria (probiotic bacteria) called lactobacilli in early infancy.

There has been much speculation over the years concerning colic and its causes. The label "colic" is often used for any baby who cries often; I prefer to use it for babies who cry for extended periods of time and are obviously experiencing stomach pain. A truly colicky baby is stiff and tense, has a distended abdomen, and has difficulty tolerating stimulation. A baby with discomfort from gas that is not so severe cries often, pulls his legs up and seems to be in pain, and may expel gas in short bursts. Often the gassy baby can be comforted by walking or rhythmic rocking and holding, while the colicky baby may or may not be comforted during an episode.

For several years I worked with a pediatric practice, specifically helping families with colicky babies. Overwhelmed by the crying, the sleepless nights, and the feelings of helplessness and incompetence, parents often said things like "My baby just doesn't like me" or "I'm just not a good parent. I can't calm him down." They were distanced from their babies instead of bonding with them. But when I could show the parents how the baby's gastrointestinal system works, and how the massage routine helps to relax the area and release painful gas, they began to understand they were doing nothing wrong as parents. I started by helping the parent to relax. Virtually every family I worked with had remarkable results within two weeks of practicing this routine every day. When parents could do the routine and get a result—that is, the baby would release gas either during the session or soon thereafter and begin to sleep for longer periods and cry less—the parents felt much more competent, began to see their babies in a more positive light, and started to bond with them again.

Massage can help any baby, from mildly gassy to extremely colicky, by stimulating the gastrointestinal system to do its job. It helps release built-up stress, and the Touch Relaxation and Resting Hands techniques help the baby learn to relax.

Colic Relief Routine

First of all, try to relax yourself. A gassy or colicky baby is a challenge for any parent, and your stress overload can make you feel edgy and confused. Remember, you are not at fault for your baby's discomfort, but you can help him. Listen to his cries with respect for his feelings, and then get to work to help him manage his episodes.

Massage the baby twice a day for two weeks, using the techniques given here. I suggest that you do this routine instead of the normal massage. That means if you have a very colicky baby who needs two weeks of twice-a-day colic relief, don't do the regular massage until after that period. In this way, the baby won't associate all massage with the discomfort that may be experienced during the Colic Relief Routine.

As you do this routine, remember to count the strokes and hold the knees-up position. Then help the baby relax with Touch Relaxation, using your voice, your hands, and rhythmic rocking, patting, and light bouncing to help him loosen up. When doing the knees-up position, do not press in too hard, just firmly; you don't want to cut off your baby's breathing!

1. RESTING HANDS

Rest your hands on your baby's tummy, relaxing yourself completely, even if the baby is fussing and crying.

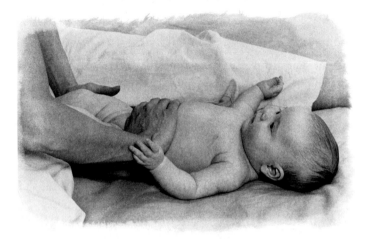

2. WATER WHEEL PART A (SEE PAGE 136)

Do this stroke six times, one hand following the other.

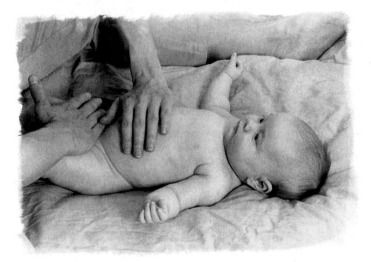

3. UP DOWN (SEE PAGE 174)

Hold the baby's knees together, then push gently up into his tummy, holding for about a half minute (count to thirty).

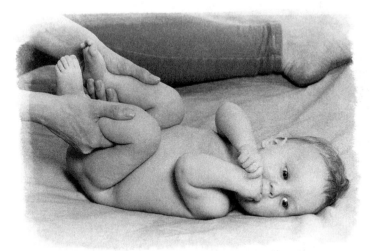

4. TOUCH RELAXATION

Gently release the pressure, stroke his legs, and use Touch Relaxation to coax him to release tension and relax.

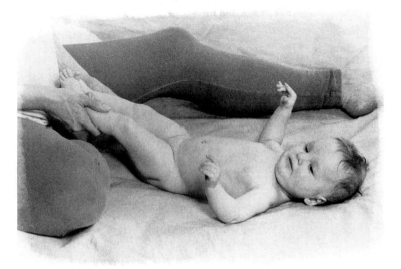

5. SUN MOON (SEE PAGE 139)

Do this stroke six times, one hand following the other.

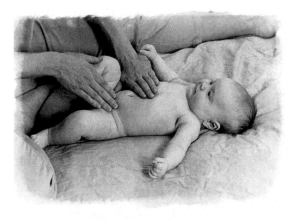

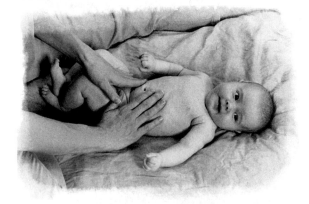

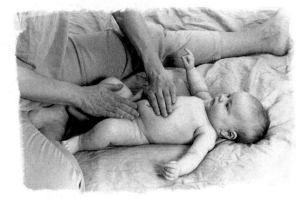

6. UP DOWN (SEE PAGE 174)

Hold the baby's knees together and push gently up into his tummy, holding for about a half minute (count to thirty).

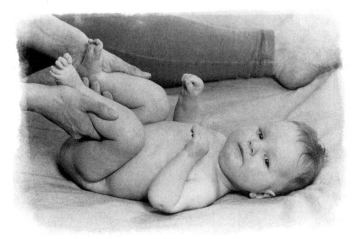

7. TOUCH RELAXATION

Gently release the pressure, stroke his legs, and use Touch Relaxation to coax him to relax and release tension.

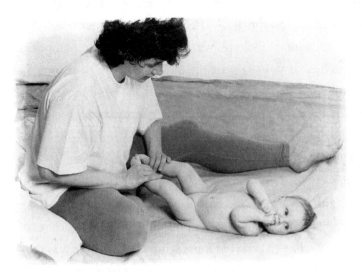

Repeat this entire cycle (steps 1 to 7) three times. It may take several days before the baby responds, and he may not expel gas on the first try. But his system will begin to function more and more smoothly, so that whenever he has an episode, a short massage will help break up and release trapped gas. Not every baby responds in the same way, and some, because of other factors, will not benefit as much as others. Still, many pediatricians now refer parents of gassy or colicky babies to infant massage instructors to address the problem without drugs.

Penny, mother of three-week-old Matthew, was nearly at the end of her rope with his colic; his pediatrician recommended she try massage, so she contacted me. When I first met Penny and Matthew, they were both so stressed by the colic that they had difficulty interacting with each other at all. "Matthew was very colicky until two weeks after I began massaging him, at which point the episodes began to subside," Penny says. "Within a few weeks, his colic disappeared completely. Now his disposition is very pleasant. He trusts me, and I have become much more relaxed." They were looking at each other and playing together, and Matthew was beginning to really enjoy being massaged. Even when Penny did the Colic Relief Routine, Matthew seemed to know how to cooperate and "work with it." With each round of strokes, he would wiggle and grunt and expel gas, and he responded well to the Touch Relaxation techniques.

Other aids may include warm baths, glycerin suppositories, and changes in diet. If you are nursing, eliminate from your own diet irritants such as tomatoes, chocolate, caffeine, and gas-producing beans and vegetables. Sometimes a milk, soy, or wheat allergy can cause colic; try eliminating one or all of these, one at a time, from your or your baby's diet, and see if there is any change in her discomfort.

Seeing your little one in such distress isn't easy, and it can be terribly draining both physically and emotionally. "Being able to massage my baby and help him relax gave me peace of mind," says Mary, mother of eighteen-month-old Michael. "I started massaging him when he was two weeks old and having painful gassy spells, and I saw results within a week. When he woke up crying in the middle of the night, I would massage him. After only a week, he would begin to relax as soon as I started stroking him. He would calm down and start releasing; often he fell asleep before I finished. I felt so good, being able to do something to help him, not to mention the extra hours of sleep it gave me! Even now, when he gets tense and out of sorts, I can talk to him and stroke him a little, and he relaxes. I wouldn't have known what to do for him otherwise. His infancy could have been just a disaster for all of us."

When my first baby was a newborn, he was very colicky. That was when I invented the Colic Relief Routine, adapting yoga techniques and advice from massage therapists to a baby's body. Within two weeks, his colic had resolved. But he remembered. When he was able to talk, he would request that I massage his tummy when he had gas pains, and he remembered to pull his knees up between strokes! This routine works for adults, too, and you may want to try it on yourself. Yoga practitioners use a similar pose, called Bhastrikasana or Bellows Pose, upon waking in the morning, as it tones the gastrointestinal system and keeps the body regularly assimilating and eliminating as it should.

Because of the incredible stress of having a colicky baby, it is natural to feel somewhat negative and discouraged. But anyone who isn't feeling well does better when lovingly touched and cared for. Your baby is no exception. Massage can be a way to help your baby and thus boost your feelings of confidence and your self-esteem. Not only will this make you a better parent, but it will help your baby feel more secure, cry less, sleep more deeply, and bond with you completely. It's worth a try.

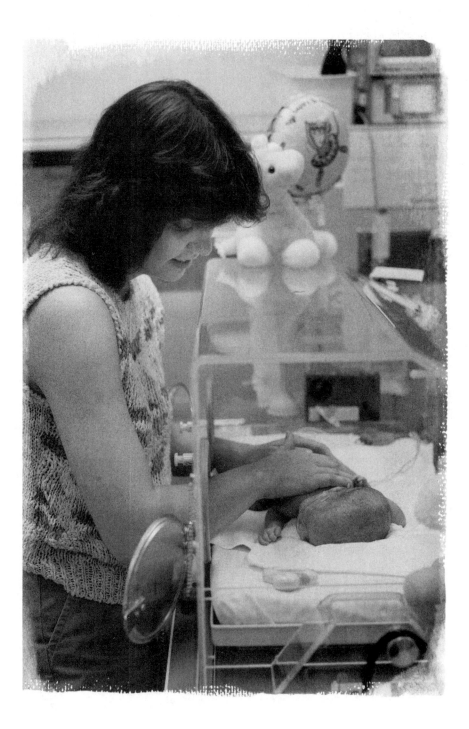

Chapter 16

Your Premature Baby

Mother, let us imagine we are traveling,
and passing through a strange
and dangerous country.

— RABINDRANATH TAGORE, "THE HERO"

Premature Babies Need a Special Kind of Touch

We know how important it is to hold our babies close, right from the start. We put a lot of planning into those first few hours and weeks, arranging to avoid the interruptions that would unnecessarily deprive our babies of those precious moments of bonding time.

When a baby arrives into the world long before she is expected, the best-laid plans are obliterated. The quiet, warm, joyous welcome hoped for is abruptly replaced by a kind of violence we never imagined. It is an unavoidable violence, one that keeps the baby alive but also engenders a tremendous range of feelings and reactions in parents.

Parents are thrust into cycles of grief, shock, denial (often manifesting as an obsession with the baby's medical condition rather than his recovery), guilt ("What did I do to cause this?"), anger (at baby, at spouse, at medical personnel, at fate), depression (often creating distance between the parent and the baby), bargaining ("I'll be the best parent ever if he just pulls through"), and fear. These feelings and many variations on them are natural and may recur in cycles for a long time after the baby's birth. Parents recover from the initial shock at different rates; most finally do accept the situation and try to find ways to help their baby through it and initiate the bonding process.

What about the premature baby? Thrust into cycles of her own—shock, pain, fear, withdrawal—she may be ignored as an emotional, feeling human being while the adults around her focus on saving her life. This kind of treatment sometimes extends far beyond what is necessary, objectifying the baby and pushing an emotional wedge between her and her parents—between her and the world.

A preemie's first contact with human touch may bring pain—needles, probes, tubes, rough handling, bright lights—suddenly, after the warm protection of the womb. One of the first things parents can do to help and to begin bonding is to touch and hold their baby. This wonderful expression of caring contributes to both physical and psychological healing, not only for babies but for parents, too. Much of the anguish of those first days and weeks can be minimized if parents can feel some sense of control.

Many studies have proven that premature babies who are regularly touched and who regularly hear their parents' voices during their nursery stay improve rapidly in growth and development. Judith Talaba, head nurse in a neonatal intensive care unit, has introduced holding methods and massage as a regular part of every baby's routine; many hospitals around the world do this now as a matter of course. "Massage gives parents a focus on the baby as an individual who needs her parents just as much as she needs the technology," Talaba says. "Parents in our nursery have become less concerned with oxygen concentrations, weight gain, and intake amounts, and more concerned about their infants being touched and massaged—a wonderful change of focus." Preemies in the Neonatal Intensive Care Unit (NICU) have responded positively to massage, she adds, losing their hyperflexia (contraction of the body) and withdrawing-from-touch behaviors. Many have also had fewer apnea (cessation of breathing) spells.

Dr. Tiffany Field has done the most extensive studies of the effects of daily massage on premature babies. Her studies have shown that when these infants were massaged every day, a number of wonderful results followed. The babies spent more time in the active alert and awake states, cried less, had lower cortisol levels (indicating less depression), and went to sleep faster after massage than they did after rocking. Over a six-week period, the massaged babies gained weight; improved on emotionality, sociability, and soothability temperament tests; had decreased urinary stress hormones; and had increased levels of serotonin (one of the brain's natural pain relievers). The babies were able to leave the hospital earlier, saving thousands of dollars for parents, hospitals, and insurance companies.

Yet another study found that snuggling with babies in the NICU eases mothers' anxiety, which can interfere with parent-child bonding.

Your Preemie in the Hospital

Preemies love the feeling of enclosure that a pair of warm, loving hands can give. But it is important to go very slowly, very tenderly. Look around your baby's environment. What changes might be made to help your baby relax and feel more comfortable, less invaded? Sometimes a small change in light, sounds, or handling can make a big difference.

A certain amount of light is necessary for the nurses to be able to observe the baby, but most nurseries will allow you to shade the baby's sensitive eyes. If your child is on a warming table, you can shield her head with an overturned box (such as a diaper box) with holes cut in all sides. In an incubator, a folded towel on top will do the trick. When the baby has stabilized, you can request that the incubator be shaded at night to help your baby regulate to cycles of day and night.

For a stark example of how our society objectifies infants, observe an adult intensive care unit and then a neonatal unit. The adult area is calm and quiet. But often the babies are subjected to loud conversation, ringing telephones, and rock music. Additional noise may include the high decibel levels of incubator monitors, the clatter of instruments and clipboards, and the slamming of incubator doors. You can ask nursery staff to lower the tone of conversation and music. You can fasten a sign on the incubator requesting gentle closing, and place a towel on top to dampen the clang of instruments.

Sounds that help your baby feel more comfortable can be introduced. Premature babies, like all babies, are soothed by their mother's voice and heartbeat sounds. When you are unable to be present, a heartbeat soother (available at many baby stores and through catalogs) may be introduced and, at intervals, a recording of your voice. First check it out with your baby; be sure the volume is low and not distressing. When you are there, talk and sing to her. Even if she doesn't seem to respond, she is listening. She remembers your voice, and it soothes her.

Your little one's first reactions to handling may be distressing. Go slowly, watch, listen, and learn from her and from sensitive hospital staff. A preemie's distress signals, which include apnea (cessation of breathing) and bradycardia (reduced heart rate), can instill so much fear that you may find yourself making excuses not to handle her.

Not surprisingly, studies show that parents are the ones who are best able to reduce their preemies' distress. Breathe deeply, relax, and move through these moments with your baby. Assure her that she is okay, that you are here to love and care for her no matter what happens. Your baby needs to feel your strength and confidence.

Observe your infant's alertness cycles to decide when the best time may be for the pre-massage techniques discussed in this chapter. Discover what kinds of stimulation she can handle. Some babies are extremely fragile and can cope with only one modality at a time—touching, talking, or eye contact, but not all three at once. Find out what kinds of drugs your baby has been given. Some (such as curare and Pavulon) will make her unresponsive. Even then, your baby is aware of you, can feel and hear you, and needs your loving touch.

Infant Massage in the NICU?

The International Association of Infant Massage is the world leader in nurturing touch, primarily due to our focus on observing cues that are in alignment with a baby's ability to receive touch. We have pioneered and refined touch concepts over decades through working with various people, including professionals in many cultures globally.

Through their cues, preemies tell you what kind of touch they are able to receive at any given moment. While the research conducted by Tiffany Field at the Touch Research Institute in Miami showed good outcomes from massaging babies in the NICU, I have come to believe that actual massage techniques are better when used after the baby is home, and that holding techniques—communication through touch—are better for premature babies.

When I first worked in a NICU, I always had the parents do the touching, not nurses, and certainly not me. I showed them Resting Hands, and how to "read" their infants to see how they were responding. IAIM now has strict policies about working with parents in the NICU, as several of our instructor trainers, with help from NICU nurses, noticed that preemies were exhibiting cues of overstimulation when massaged.

One review concludes that there seems to be an increase in weight gain in infants receiving regular massage, and some reduction in length of hospital stay (likely linked to the increased weight gain), but little evidence of other beneficial outcomes. While the evidence that regular massage leads to increased weight gain is good, your baby has many more important needs than that; trained observation of how your tiny one is receiving stimuli is important before adding more stimuli to his day.

Cherry Bond, a neonatal nurse and IAIM Certified Infant Massage Instructor, developed the 5-Step Dialogue, which helps parents to do something *with* their babies rather than *to* their babies. She says, "Every cue is like a single word in a sentence, which is part of a whole story that parents can use to participate in a unique dialogue with their baby." Certified Infant Massage Instructors with IAIM can help parents through this

5-Step Dialogue, which includes how to observe babies' cues, how to understand the concept of permission, and various ways to touch and hold the baby.

After your preemie is home from the hospital and can be considered a newborn, you can begin to practice the art of infant massage. I suggest that you attend a class after reading this book. In the back, under "Resources," you can find the websites of IAIM, where you can find an instructor in your area.

How to Begin

You can begin your baby's massage routine with a simple daily dose of warm touch, the Resting Hands. This method is best while your baby is hospitalized; you can begin regular massage strokes when you bring him home from the hospital. Hold his tiny body in cupped hands, with a feeling of heaviness and deep relaxation in your hands. Practice your Controlled Belly Breathing. Feel relaxation and warmth in your hands. Respect your baby's communication, however subtle it may be. Watch for cues so you know when he needs a break from any stimulation.

Conveying respect is an important part of infant massage. While he is forming initial feelings about himself and his body, whatever you reflect back to him will be taken seriously.

Kangaroo Care

Kangaroo care is now being used in NICUs everywhere. The idea is for parents to hold their infants on their chests—ideally, skin-to-skin. With infants who need a lot of medical intervention, this can be difficult, but not impossible. Nurses can help you place your baby on your chest, with whatever tubes and wires are connected to her.

Research confirms that secure bonds between parents and infants are critical to healthy development for children. For infants that are born prematurely, bonding may be interrupted by the complexity of life in the NICU. A study at a large NICU, presented at the American Academy of Pediatrics National Conference and Exhibition in 2015, shows that a little skin-to-skin snuggling between parents and infants can decrease parental stress. The study examined mothers' stress levels before and after they held their babies kangaroo style (skin-to-skin inside the pouch of the parent's shirt) for at least one hour.

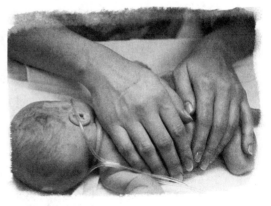

"We found that all of the mothers reported an objective decrease in their stress level after skin-to-skin contact with their babies," says neonatologist Natalia Isaza, M.D., F.A.A.P., of Children's National Health System in Washington, D.C. This was especially true regarding the reported stress of being separated from their infants, feeling helpless and unable to protect their infant from pain and painful procedures, and the general experience in the NICU, she says.

"We already know there are physiological benefits in the newborns when they are held skin to skin," Dr. Isaza says, such as stabilization of heart rate, breathing patterns, and blood-oxygen levels, gains in sleep time and weight, decreased crying, greater breastfeeding success, and earlier hospital discharge. "Now we have more evidence that skin-to-skin contact can also decrease parental stress that can interfere with bonding, health and emotional wellness, and the interpersonal relations of parents, as well as breastfeeding rates. This is a simple technique to benefit both parent and child that perhaps should be encouraged in all NICUs."

Parents who sing to their preemies during kangaroo care can improve both their infant's health and their own. An *Acta Pediatrica* study of eighty-six mother-infant pairs in a NICU in Meir Hospital in Israel confirmed this idea. It compared preemies whose mothers held them skin-to-skin but did not sing with infants whose mothers held them and sang to

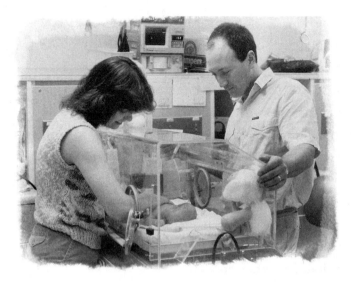

them. The second group had improved heart rate variability patterns. The combined effect of kangaroo care and singing also helped mothers to feel less anxiety. Lead author Dr. Shmuel Arnon said, "We recommend combining kangaroo care and maternal singing for stable preterm infants. These safe, inexpensive, and easily implemented therapies can be applied during daily neonatal care."

Eye Contact

A powerful connection is made when your baby first looks into your eyes. Eye contact is one of the important components in the dance of bonding and one of the joys of massage. But preemies, because they are not yet ready to regulate themselves, need your help. Your baby may avoid eye contact altogether. You can gently offer encouragement by reducing harsh lights and positioning the baby so that you are accessible. Or your baby may become "locked in"—unable to release herself from looking and eventually becoming overstressed. If this happens, you can gently unlock her gaze by moving aside, passing a hand in front of her face, or shifting her position.

As your baby grows, her ability to communicate with you through eye contact will grow. Be patient, and don't force it. With slow and steady encouragement, you will soon treasure this important part of your bond.

Trouble Spots

Premature babies' bodies have been traumatized. Observe which areas of your baby's body may be especially programmed for pain. Often the feet, head, and chest are quite sensitive. Observe your baby and his cues.

Using Resting Hands in the NICU

1. Place your hands around your baby's body, cupping her body within your hands.
2. Deeply relax all over, taking several belly breaths. Let this relaxation move from your heart through your arms and hands and to your baby.
3. Observe your baby for cues and talk to her. Acknowledge that she has had a lot of pain and that she has been very brave. You are here to help her release the pain and let pleasure in. Let her know that soon this painful time will be over, and she will be healthy and happy, ready to do what she wants to do in life.
4. If your baby is not showing any stress cues, move your hands to cover her body. Again, allow relaxation to move from your heart through your arms and hands and to your baby. Talk to her and with her, responding to what she may be communicating to you: "Are there too many things that are stimulating? Is it too noisy or too bright? What can I do to help you?"
5. If your baby responds with relaxation, praise her effort.
6. When the baby is ready, have the nurses help you to place her on your chest, perhaps as you sit in a rocking chair.

Stress Cues

Some researchers have found that babies in intensive care give cues to indicate they are stressed out. These cues tend to be universal; these may not all apply to your baby, so use the nurses' knowledge and your own intuition and observation to let you know what applies to your baby and when. These cues can include skin mottling, hiccups, gagging, apnea, bradycardia, and gestures of turning away or raising a hand in front of the face as if she is warding off incoming stimuli.

These signs do not mean you should stop Resting Hands altogether. Give her a break and try again at another time. If your baby continues to show signs of distress, let her sleep, and try again later. Remember to breathe deeply and relax, and do not allow anyone to make you feel incompetent to care for your baby. Gradually your baby's stimulation threshold will rise, and you will be able to touch and then massage her when she gets home.

Massaging Your Premature Baby at Home

You can really begin to work with your baby when he comes home from the hospital. Keep in mind that it is quite a change for him and that he may regress a little. You may have to back up a bit with the massage, again focusing on Resting Hands, relaxation, and release.

In the warmth and security of your home environment, your baby will at last be able to release the tension and trauma of the hospital stay. This can be frightening and difficult for parents; suddenly the baby may be crying all the time. You may feel a little insecure without the hospital staff, as much as you may have previously resented their intrusions. At a time when you need reassurance, your baby's feedback seems to be "I don't like it here!"

Actually, the intense crying, if not caused by pain, is a healthy release. Often a baby will cry especially hard after a massage. This does not mean that he dislikes it or that you are doing it incorrectly. It is simply the only way available to him to release all his pent-up anguish. You can support your child by trying to relax and allow him to do what he needs to do, by being there to lovingly comfort him, and by trying to release your own fears. If you feel like crying with the baby (who wouldn't?), go right ahead.

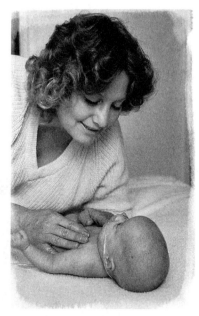

Eventually you will progress from simple relaxation and holding to massage. Still, there are differences between massaging a premature baby and massaging a full-term infant. Begin by massaging the place on the baby's body that has been least invaded—usually the back. Miniaturize every stroke. Follow the strokes in Chapter 13, and simply modify them; for example, use two or three fingers instead of the whole hand. But do not be afraid to be firm. Your baby loves to feel the strength of your presence; a feathery touch can be overstimulating and irritating.

Be sure the space is very warm and that the baby is enclosed (use the Cradle Pose, or support the baby with firm pillows) and near you. You may want to warm the oil beforehand, but swishing it between your palms should be sufficient. Soon just the sound of the oil between your palms will cause your baby to open up like a little flower. He will learn to anticipate being massaged as a pleasurable experience, a time to feel the security of your loving hands. Once the tension is out of his body, his system will regulate. You will find marked improvement in his sleeping, feeding, digestion, and elimination, and you will notice a decrease in crying. Watch your baby bloom, open to acceptance of life.

If possible, schedule yourself for an all-body massage by a competent, licensed therapist. You, too, have been through quite an ordeal. If you can relieve your own tensions and trauma, your baby will respond more positively to your touch.

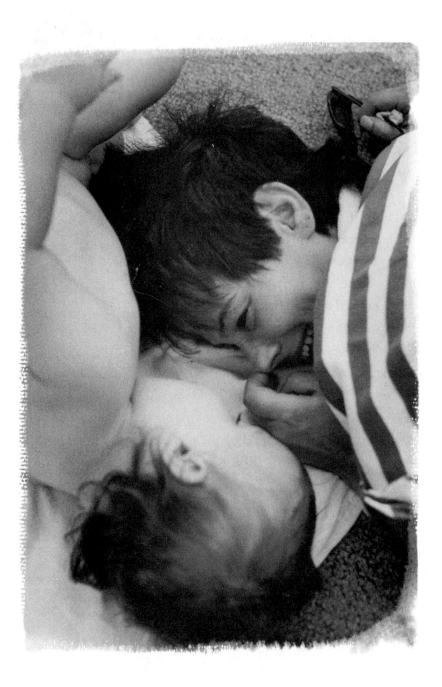

Chapter 17

Your Baby with Special Needs

The neighbor calls him a mongoloid.
The doctor says Down syndrome.
I call him Kim.

—MIA ELMSATER, CERTIFIED INFANT
MASSAGE INSTRUCTOR TRAINER

Bonding and Attachment with Special Babies

Bonding is a matter of reciprocal interaction. It depends upon a parent stimulating the infant with appropriate cues or signals, that trigger a response in the infant. The infant's cues or signals then trigger further involvement by the parent, including eye contact, smiling, speech sounds, and body movements. The baby with mental, visual, hearing, or developmental impairments or delays sometimes cannot respond in the ordinary manner to parental cues. Interactional synchrony thus may be inhibited, which can lead to the parent feeling out of touch with her baby. In addition, parents of babies with special needs are often overwhelmed by all of the information they need to absorb, by the therapies they are expected to carry out, and by the double bind of grieving and celebrating a new baby at the same time.

Parents' emotional reactions to the discovery of a special need in their newborn differ greatly. They can include confusion, denial, guilt, anger, wishful thinking, depression, intellectualization, and acceptance. These natural feelings can overlap and recur as parent and child adjust to their life together and to each new stage of the baby's development.

Infant massage can be a wonderful bonding tool for parents and babies with special needs. While physiological benefits do accrue, the focus and goal of infant massage are the interaction and connection of these two people. It is something you do *with* your baby rather than *to* your baby. It is not another therapy but an opportunity to share your love. A daily massage connects parent and baby in a way that no other type of interaction can match. Babies with special needs benefit from this intimacy even more than other babies. Because some avenues of communication may not be open to them, their parents need to know them well: the way the body feels when tense or relaxed, the look and feel of the abdomen when gassy or not, the difference between pain and tension. Often such parents need to be acutely aware of their infants' bodies because life-threatening infections can arise. A parent who is attuned to the look and feel of her baby's body at all times will more likely be able to detect toxicity in the early stages.

Elizabeth has cystic fibrosis, and her mother is glad she learned infant massage when Elizabeth was an infant. "At first we didn't massage our baby every day," Elizabeth's mother says, "but the more we did it and saw how wonderfully she responded, it grew on us. Elizabeth doesn't have her problem with being cold anymore. (If she does, we give her a massage.) She does not have so much abdominal pain, and her whole body is relaxed. Now when we massage Elizabeth, we concentrate not so much on cystic fibrosis as on Elizabeth as a beautiful little human being, a person. Infant massage has helped us have a relationship with her that has gone beyond our expectations. . . . It gives us great hope."

In this chapter, we will be discussing some particular challenges and how the massage may be altered for various types of conditions. Of course, this chapter cannot tell you how to best use massage with your baby in various challenging situations, since there are just too many types of challenges, and within those categories many different babies with varying needs. What I can do, however, is give you some general information and hints to start with, so you then can approach your baby's physician, occupational therapist, or physical therapist with a basic knowledge of infant massage.

Before beginning a massage routine with your baby, check with the baby's doctor and physical therapist. They will help you design the massage and relaxation to suit your baby's needs. The International Association of Infant Massage offers continuing education programs for Certified Infant Massage Instructors (CIMIs) who work with babies who have medical challenges. I encourage you to seek out a CIMI with this extra knowledge to help you work with caregivers to massage your special baby.

Then trust yourself. You know your child better than anyone else. You are his or her specialist, and a companion in a way no one else ever can be.

Developmental Challenges

Developmental challenges such as cerebral palsy manifest in many different ways. The child's physical therapist will use procedures that either inhibit (relax) or facilitate (stimulate) muscle tone. Inhibitory techniques may include slow stroking, gentle shaking, positioning, rocking, and neutral warmth. Facilitating techniques may include icing, brushing, positioning, pressure, and vibration. The massage strokes in this book can be modified to either inhibit or facilitate. To inhibit, use long, slow, sweeping strokes and Touch Relaxation; to facilitate, use a more vigorous stroking and more playful interactions such as bouncy rhymes and songs.

The massage can be delivered in the same sequence as the massage in Chapter 13, with the following changes:

- Stroking the bottom of the foot often causes a reaction of extension and tightening of the leg. If this occurs in Under Toes, Ball of Foot, and Thumb Press, change the stroke so that pressure is exerted on the outside rather than on the balls of the feet.

- The Thumbs to Sides stroke on the tummy is particularly helpful in improving and stimulating diaphragmatic breathing.
- Infants with developmental challenges often show signs of resistance when the shoulders are stroked. For the chest, begin with Resting Hands, then try just one stroke, such as the Butterfly stroke across the chest, which includes the shoulder, and gradually increase as the child's stimulation threshold rises.
- For the face, the Smile strokes aid lip closure to promote good swallowing. These are particularly good for babies who drool and breathe through the mouth. The facial massage is an excellent prelude to oral stimulation and feeding therapy for the child who is sensitive around the mouth.
- When doing the Colic Relief Routine, do not hold the knees against the stomach for more than a count of five, so as not to inhibit respiration.

Babies who are tactile defensive—that is, hypersensitive and reactive to skin contact—benefit from firm pressure and stroking. Warm baths and brisk rubbing with a terry-cloth towel before massage can increase acceptance of skin-to-skin massage.

According to cerebral palsy experts, a slow, firm stroke down the center of the back can increase brain organization. Do not stroke up the back against hair growth.

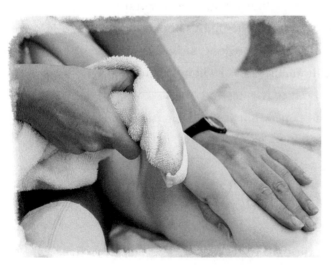

If your baby has a shunt or other type of bypass, her physical therapist will be able to tell you how much pressure is appropriate and how to work around these areas, even if at first the only thing you can do is use the Resting Hands technique on another part of the body such as the legs.

If your baby has had surgery, you can use massage, holding techniques, and Touch Relaxation with other parts of his body, with the support of his physician. Your loving touch and the security of it can be very important to your baby's recovery.

Visual Challenges

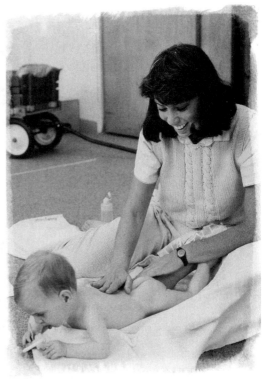

Massage can be a particularly positive experience for babies with visual challenges because of their need for tactile stimulation as a means to define their world. Researchers have found remarkable results in both animal and human babies with visual challenges when tactile stimulation is used. One study reported that visual impairment did not produce a depression of emotional and learning behavior in animals if they received touch stimulation, whereas if this touch stimulation was withdrawn, they became either excessively passive or hyperaggressive. Infants with visual challenges whose parents are particularly effective in establishing emotional bonds with them show a great deal of social interaction, perceptual attentiveness, and responsiveness in the first few months of life. These babies are able to reach toward sounds earlier than other babies with visual impairments.

Massage helps babies form an effective body image; this is important in establishing the object constancy that allows the baby to let go of the parent and begin exploring the environment. In babies with visual challenges, motor development in the first few months is not different from that of babies with full sight, although there is often a lag in the onset of crawling and walking. Some researchers suggest that this may be due to the blind infant's resistance to lying prone (facedown), which may curtail

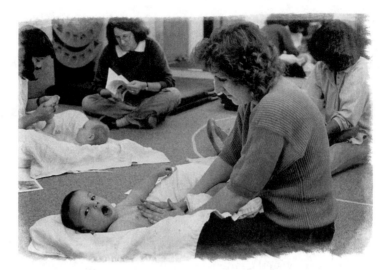

the development of upper body strength, which is necessary for reaching and crawling. Massage in the prone position may gradually help the baby accept this position for play because massage becomes associated with trust and safety.

Your voice and touch simultaneously communicate love to your baby. Because you may not get the facial response you instinctively expect, you may find yourself withdrawing. Instead, find ways to develop an intimate rapport with your child through touch. Talk to your baby during the massage, explaining what you are doing and telling her what will happen next. Use her name often, and exaggerate auditory cues such as swishing the oil between your palms. During the first six months, do not use music or other sounds besides your voice. Later, music that imitates the rhythm of the strokes can be used as long as you interact with the music in a way that connects it to the massage, such as by singing or humming along and stroking your baby to the music. Keep your face close, and always keep one hand on his body. Always begin the massage with auditory cues and by gently holding and stroking the baby's legs and feet to initiate contact. Consider the light source during the massage. Light can be distracting to some babies with partial vision, while others need a stronger light source to feel comfortable.

I recommend getting the CDs of our signature lullaby, "Ami Tomake Bhalobashi Baby" (Chapter 11). One CD has the lullaby with beautiful music, sung by a woman with an exquisite voice; the other CD has just the music. See InfantMassageWarehouse.com and AmiTomake.com.

Auditory Challenges

Babies with hearing challenges have the same need for tactile comfort as other babies. Affectionate interaction is the most important element in any baby's life. Babies with auditory challenges need to be spoken to. During this early period, sound stimulates the growth of nerve connections between the baby's ear and brain. The sound stimulation in every baby's world creates an evolving network of nerve pathways. Many babies with hearing challenges are fitted with hearing aids to increase the amount of sound stimulation they receive. You can keep these on during the massage. The organization Infant Hearing Resource makes recommendations that might well be applied to all babies: "Tell the baby what you are thinking and feeling. He likes to hear about what makes you feel happy, sad, anxious, and excited. He can tell from the way you hold him and from your body language that you are experiencing different feelings. Then, when he has different feelings, he will know what to call them."

Use normal speech with your baby during massage time, and make relaxed and loving eye contact with him as much as possible. Describe what you are doing. For example: "This is your foot, Jason. And here are your toes. One, two, three, four, five toes!" Converse with your baby and imitate his sounds. Experts agree that "parentese" or baby talk is a perfectly normal and acceptable form of communication with babies who have auditory challenges. Parents who choose to learn and teach sign language can begin during the massage, even before the baby can indicate comprehension of the signs.

Massaging Babies with Serious Medical Conditions

The Touch Research Institute is continually replicating studies that prove that babies who have every imaginable problem—prematurity, HIV, cocaine exposure, depressed mothers, sexual and physical abuse, asthma, autism, diabetes, rheumatoid arthritis, developmental delays, eating disorders, dermatitis, cancer, burns, and post-traumatic stress disorder—all benefit from loving touch and massage. Massage in these cases has resulted in lower anxiety and stress hormones, and improved scores on all clinical scoring methods.

Generally, special precautions must be taken when massaging these babies, and the nursing staff can help you learn about these. Work with your baby's nurses, suggesting holding techniques such as Resting Hands, carrying such as kangaroo care, and massage. If they don't know, contact your local Certified Infant Massage Instructor with IAIM. If she or he does not have special training in this area, request that he or she find an instructor trainer who is familiar with this field and get the information you need. The references at the end of this book may help you, too. Remember, you are the parent. You have the right to research and discover healthy ways to establish a strong bond with your baby.

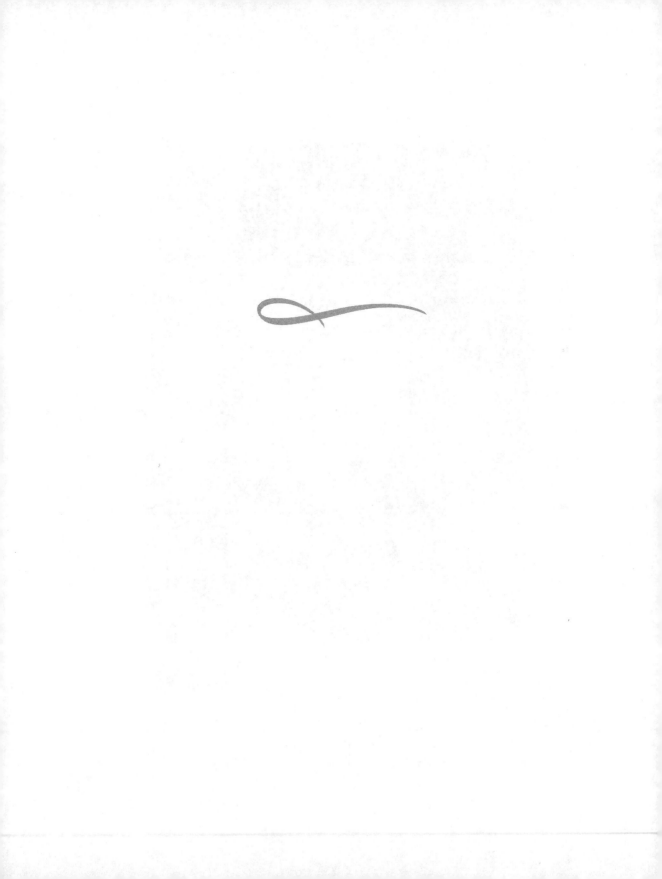

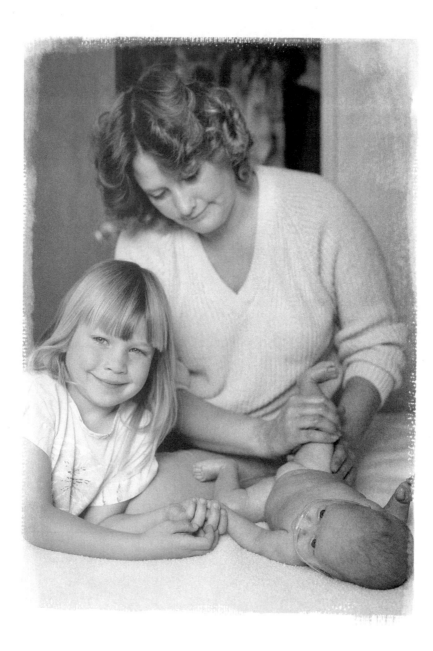

Chapter 18

Your Growing Child and Sibling Bonding Through Massage

The plant's bright blessings
Spring forth
From Earth's gentle being,
And human children rise up
With grateful hearts to join
the spirits of the world.

—RUDOLF STEINER

Big Kids Need Touching, Too

One evening after a family gathering at which a newborn cousin had made his first appearance, a friend's six-year-old daughter climbed into her mother's lap. "I wish I was a baby, Mommy," she said, "then I'd get a lot of attention." That was a signal—time for a bedtime massage. Why? Not so much because she needed more attention, but because she needed to talk about the feelings her new cousin stirred in her.

It is important for children to talk about their feelings, but sometimes it is difficult to get them to open up. Often the more we question, the more unresponsive they become. My eight-year-old was to have surgery within a week, and though I knew he should talk about his fears, I hadn't yet been able to draw him out. The day after we had taken a tour of the chil-

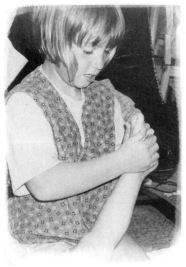

dren's ward and met the nurses at the hospital, he mumbled, shrugged his shoulders, and slunk off to his room.

Later that evening I offered him a foot massage. I gently massaged his calves, knees, and feet; within five minutes he relaxed and began to talk. He had several questions about the hospital and his surgery and was finally able to get the reassurance he needed—that I would be there with him, that he would not wake up during the surgery, and that he would be able to talk after his tonsillectomy. The operation went smoothly, and I remembered to use the soothing power of touch with him throughout the experience, before and after the surgery. A foot or hand massage now and then helped us both relax and let go of scary feelings.

Anthropologist Ashley Montagu, author of *Touching,* states that a child's close relationship with his parents is a source of basic self-esteem. "Persons who are callously unresponsive to human need, who have become so hardened that they are no longer in touch with the human condition, are not merely metaphorically so," he says, "but clearly physiologically so." A study reported in the *Journal of Humanistic Psychology* confirmed this idea, indicating that the higher the subject's self-esteem, the more he communicates through touch. Before the age of twelve, children are more tactile-kinesthetic—that is, they use feeling more than sight or hearing for information about the world. Therefore, a warm touch can often trigger an outpouring of feeling or thoughts more than verbal communication. Saying "I love you" to your child is important, but more important is communicating your love through eye contact, through focused attention, and through your loving touch. In addition, for children, when praise is accompanied by touch, it is believed and absorbed 85 percent of the time, whereas praise given only with words is taken in only 15 percent of the time.

Bonding between parents and children continues as the children age. Simply because a child has graduated from the in-arms stage doesn't mean she no longer needs your attention through healthy touching. She will no longer be nursing, she won't cuddle in the same way, her circle of support will widen, and she will be increasingly busy exploring the infinite possibilities of her world. But as she grows out of her mother's and father's arms, she will come to cherish those moments of closeness that reassure her that Mommy and Daddy are always there with a warm smile and a loving massage.

According to Ashley Soderlund, Ph.D., in an article titled "What Is the First Sensory System to Develop in Babies?," "connecting through touch with older babies and toddlers promotes bonding and secure attachment. Hugs can comfort a sad or scared child, and massages can help an overly tired child calm down. Giving a toddler a massage fifteen minutes before bedtime has been shown to reduce sleep problems, according to a study published in August 2001 in *Early Child Development and Care.* The sense of touch in a newborn is a powerful tool for connection, calming and nurturing development."

Though sometime in the first nine months is the ideal time to start the massage routine, it is never too late to begin. Usually a child between one and three years of age who has not been massaged from infancy will be much too busy to be still, but you may be able to start with a short, gentle back rub at bedtime. When the child becomes accustomed to being massaged, he will begin to ask for it. Before you know it, he is massaging you!

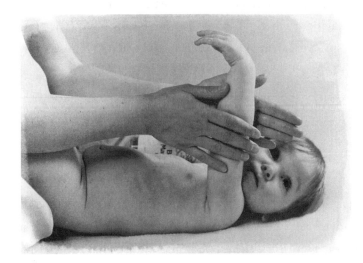

How to Begin

Perhaps you've never considered massage as a means of opening communication between you and your child. How do you start without making it a big deal? The Soccer Player's Special (or Ballerina's Special—whatever suits the child's interests) is a good way to begin. Here's how:

1. Make sure the area is warm and comfortable with no distractions.
2. Wash your hands and remove jewelry.
3. Bedtime or after a bath is a good time, when your child is clean and ready to relax.
4. Always begin by asking permission, and respect your child's choices. Even when you move to another body part, you can say, "May I massage your tummy now?"
5. Use a natural oil, just enough to make your movements smooth without excessive oil.
6. Massage one leg at a time. Use the Milking and Rolling strokes (Chapter 13). Use your thumbs to work circles around the knees, your fingertips to gently massage calf muscles, your thumbs to work all over the feet.
7. Build self-esteem by saying positive things about your child while massaging, such as "You have such beautiful hair," or "I noticed you shared your toys with your friend today. That was very nice of you. You are such a generous person."

Ages and Stages for Massage

At different stages, your child will respond to being massaged differently. My best advice is to go with the flow, allowing her to lead you in the appropriate way. Here are some very common stages that children go through with massage, and suggestions about what to do when your baby begins to respond differently. Of course, these ages are not rigid; each child will have his own rhythm and cycles of growth.

The Active Crawler

Active crawling is a challenging time for most parents, who are accustomed to the time they spend massaging their infant as a soothing, quiet, communicative, and even meditative experience. When your baby starts crawling, massage becomes more playful and fun. Just about anything is preferable to lying on her back! You can use rhymes and games, or give her a toy to play with or a hard biscuit to suck on. Instead of adhering rigidly to the sequence of stroking, just massage the part that appears in front of you. Babies will roll around, crawl, climb into your lap, sit up, and do all manner of movements. Be creative with your massage. My son and I made a game; he would start to crawl away, and I would say, "Oh, no you don't! I'm gonna get you now!" and laugh, pulling him back toward my lap. He would giggle and want to do this over and over again. In the meantime, I massaged his back, his buttocks, and his legs and feet.

The Toddler

From ages one to three, your child will be developing her autonomy, and a big part of autonomy is exercising her freedom to say no. She may often reject massage altogether during this period. If this is her response when you offer a massage, respect her choice. Sometimes she may ask for massage in a coded way, such as "I have a tummyache." Then you can offer a massage. You can do the strokes in a playful way. Clara Ute Zacher Laves, an IAIM Instructor Trainer, suggests doing fun things like pretending to plant a garden on your child's back or make a pizza on her tummy. Use your imagination, and your child will enjoy this opportunity for creative play. The Milking strokes should be done in two parts: first the thigh (or upper arm) and then the calf (or forearm). The Hug and Glide stroke and the Rolling stroke should start just below the knee or elbow rather than the hip or shoulder, to prevent twisting the joint.

The Preschool Child

At about age three, your child will settle down and enjoy being massaged again in a more quiet way. Now that he has established his independence, he will like the feeling of being a "baby" again, receiving all of his parent's attention. You can massage after a bath or at bedtime. Adapt the strokes to the child's growing limbs, leaving out strokes that don't fit or seem appropriate. Respect the modesty your child may have developed by now, and allow him to keep his T-shirt and underwear on. Tell a story as you massage legs, feet, tummy, and back, or ask your child what body part you are massaging, helping him to learn the names of different parts, such as forearm, thigh, calf, and so on. From now on, you can leave out the Gentle Movements, as your child is getting plenty of stretching and exercise in his day-to-day life.

The School-Age Child

Again, you will adapt the strokes to your child's growing limbs, kneading the thigh and calf muscles as she lies flat rather than using the Milking stroke or the Hug and Glide stroke. Offer open-ended questions or statements that will encourage her to talk, such as "It seemed like you were a little sad when you came home today." Music, storytelling, and talking can enhance the massage experience and allow time for your child to feel special and open up to you. You might add scent to your massage oil, allowing her to choose the scent. Most school-age children will enjoy the massage more if they are lying on their stomach rather than face-up.

The Massage in Schools Program

An exciting development has come out of the more than thirty years that the International Association of Infant Massage has been incorporated. Mia Elmsater and Sylvie Hetu, both Senior International Trainers for IAIM, combined their experience with infant massage with knowledge about tactile stimulation for children and adults with special needs and with information about massage, play, and touch therapy. They founded a new movement and organization called the Massage in Schools Association (MISA). MISA International has two main categories of affiliated members: the Massage in Schools Program (MISP) trainers and the MISA-affiliated branches. They believe in the principle that a shared core curriculum as a solid base is necessary for a program to be successful. Their ultimate vision is that there will be thousands of MISA instructors and hundreds of MISP trainers, all teaching the program, all sharing their dedication with love so that the nurturing touch will become a way of life for children in all schools worldwide. Using massage in schools is a new concept in modern-day society. Although massage, especially as it is practiced in some native and traditional cultures, is as old as mankind itself, it is only in the past century that science has been able to explain the benefits of massage.

When they put this program together, Elmsater and Hetu discussed in depth which ages would be suitable. The study of child development as well as their respective experiences in preschool, day care centers, and schools led them to the range of four to twelve years old. So far the program has had great success for children as well as for their parents and teachers. Children doing the simple routine lower their stress levels, increasing the chances that they will concentrate better at school and sleep better at home. For more information about MISA, see their website, massageinschools.com. Another website that has great information about MISP and infant massage is journeywithjash.com.

The Adolescent

With adolescents, it is often hard to give a massage, as self-consciousness is high during this period. You can offer a foot or back massage as you talk to your child about his day. If he is open, you can then offer, "Would you like me to rub your calves?" During this period, stay away from body parts associated with sexuality, as your child will be uncomfortable with this, and it is appropriate to keep boundaries intact as he grows into adulthood. Again, your adolescent will enjoy the massage more if he is lying on his stomach as opposed to face-up. Offer pillows under the stomach or other areas for comfort.

When your daughter begins menstruation, if she has cramps, you can massage her belly or lower back to ease her discomfort. Using the heel of your palm, push up the lower back at the tailbone to relieve cramps and pressure. Acupressure points at the Achilles tendon, just under either side of the ankle bone, can be massaged, which often relieves cramping. You can have her sit up on the floor between your knees and knead tension from her neck and shoulders as you talk about whatever is on her mind. With her face turned away from you, it is easier for her to talk about feelings and worries.

Rhymes and Games for the Older Baby

Massaging an older baby requires a different approach from massaging an infant. To keep the child interested and involved, you may want to vary the massage each time, adding stories, songs, and animation. For example, one of the tummy strokes most enjoyed by toddlers is I Love You (Chapter 13). They enjoy chiming in with you as you stretch your words out, cooing in a singsong voice. When you massage the feet, you can recite "This Little Piggy." Little games, songs, and stories that you invent as you massage your little one will involve him, entertain his alive mind, and promote the kind of communication that stimulates and utilizes all of his developing senses.

Feet and Toes
This little piggy went to market
This little piggy stayed home
This little piggy had roast beef *[tofu? pomegranates?]*
This little piggy had none
This little piggy went wee wee wee all the way home.

One is a lady that sits in the sun;
Two is a baby, and three is a nun;

Four is a lily with innocent breast;
Five is a birdie asleep in his nest.

This little piggy got into the barn.
This one ate all the corn.
This one said he wasn't well,
This one said he'd go and tell,
And this one said—squeak, squeak, squeak!
"I can't get over the barn door sill!"

See saw, Marjorie Daw,
The hen flew over the barn.
She counted her baby chicks one by one,
    [Count each toe except the baby toe]
But she couldn't find the little brown [white] one.

    [Start with the little toe]
This little cow eats grass,
This little cow eats hay,
This little cow looks over the hedge,
This little cow runs away,
And this *big* cow does nothing at all
But lie in the fields all day!
We'll chase her, and chase her,
And chase her!

    [This rhyme goes well with the foot strokes using thumbs
    that press all over the foot]
Pitty patty polt,
Shoe the wild colt.
Here a nail,
And there a nail,
Pitty patty polt!

Tummy

[Use this rhyme with the Sun Moon stroke]

Round and round the garden

Went the teddy bear,

One step, two step, tickle under there!

[Walk fingers up to armpit]

Fingers

Five little fishes swimming in a pool

[Open hand]

First one said, "The pool is cool."

Second one said, "The pool is deep."

Third one said, "I want to sleep."

Fourth one said, "Let's dive and dip."

Fifth one said, "I spy a ship."

They all jumped up and went ker-splash

[Stroke top of hand]

Away the five little fishes dash.

[Gently wiggle hand to relax]

[Begin with thumb]

This is the father, short and stout.

This is the mother, with children all about.

This is the brother, tall you see.

This is the sister with dolly on her knee.

This is the baby, sure to grow.

And here is the family, all in a row.

Here is a tree with leaves so green,

Here are the apples that hang between

[Hold baby's thumb and small finger and dangle three middle fingers]

When the wind blows the apples fall

[Hold baby's wrist and gently wiggle]

And here is a basket to gather them all.
  [Cup baby's hand in yours]

Five little kittens
All black and white
  [Cup baby's fist in your hands]
Sleeping soundly
All through the night
Meow, meow, meow, meow, meow
  [Raise each finger]
It's time to get up now!

Within a little apple
So cozy and so small
There are five little chambers
  [Cup baby's fist in yours]
Around a little hall.
In every room are sleeping
Two seeds of golden brown
They're lying there and dreaming
  [Open each finger and peek in]
In beds of eiderdown.
They're dreaming there of sunshine
And how it's going to be
  [Stroke top of hand]
When they shall hang as apples
Upon the Christmas tree.
  [Hold baby's wrist and gently wiggle]

Face
Knock knock
  [Open Book stroke on forehead]

Peek in
   [Gently open eyes with thumbs]
Open the latch
   [With thumbs, push up on the bridge of nose and draw diagonally
   across cheeks—"Happy Sinuses and Cheek Muscles"]
And walk right in.
   [Smile strokes]
Hello, Mr. Chinny-chin-chin!
   [Gently wiggle chin]

Two little eyes to look around
Two little ears to hear each sound
One little nose to smell what's sweet
One little mouth that likes to eat.

Peek-a-boo, I see you
Hiding behind the chair
Peek-a-boo, I see you
Hiding there.

Games to Play with Gentle Movements

Arms
Up so high
   [Stretch arms up]
Down so low
   [Bring arms down]
Give a little shake
   [Wiggle hands at wrist]
And hold them so.
   [Put palms together]

This is my right arm, hold it flat

[Hold right arm out to the side, flat on surface]

This is my left arm, just like that.

[Repeat with left arm]

Right arm

[Bring right arm across chest]

Left arm

[Bring left arm across chest to hug self]

Hug myself!

Left arm

[Open out left arm]

Right arm

[Repeat with right arm]

Catch a little elf!

[Bring palms together quickly, then ask, "Did you catch him?" and peek in cupped hands]

Pat-a-cake, pat-a-cake

[Clap baby's hands together]

Baker man,

Bake me a cake as fast as you can.

[Hold arms up, then down]

Roll it

[Roll hands around each other]

And pat it

[Pat palms together]

And mark it with a B

[Make a B with baby's hand]

And put it in the oven

[Hold arms up, then down]

For baby and me.

[Point to baby and self]

Legs

One leg, two legs

  [Cross legs over tummy, right leg on top]

Hot cross buns

  [Cross legs over tummy, left leg on top]

Right leg, left leg

  [Pull legs gently toward you, flat on surface]

Isn't that fun?

  [Gently wiggle legs to release tension]

Up

  [Knees into tummy]

Down

  [Gently pull legs out straight]

Up

  [Knees into tummy]

Down

  [Gently pull legs out straight]

And shake them all around.

  [Gently wiggle legs to release tension]

Helping an Older Child Adjust to a New Baby

A new baby is a fascinating, fearful creature to her older sibling. Hovered over and protected by adults, she seems an unapproachable, somehow dangerous little thing. Much has been written on the importance of letting your older child know that he is still loved and cherished in his own right when a new baby comes into the family. The next step is to help the older child and the baby begin a relationship of their own. It usually takes quite a bit longer for a child to fully bond with a new sibling. His first task is to understand that the baby is "here," that mother is all right, that he is still loved as much as before, and that life goes on.

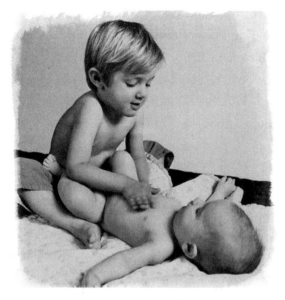

As you massage your baby every day, your older child will observe. He may remember being massaged (in fact, he still may enjoy being massaged) and identify with the baby. They share an experience and have something in common. If you give your child the opportunity to massage the baby occasionally (only if he wants to, of course), he will benefit by it in many ways, as will the baby. The older child will bond with the baby in the same ways that you do—with eye contact, touch, movement, and sound. He will learn that the baby is not necessarily so dangerous and fragile but a person like himself. His confidence will bloom as he comes to realize his own competence as a caregiver and protector. The baby will respond to him, overcoming her initial fear of his sometimes clumsy or rough handling or his startling behavior. She will begin to relate to him as a loving peer and ally.

It is best to delay suggesting that an older child massage the new baby until the baby has passed through that stage of fragility when she is easily startled. Usually three or four months of age is about the right time, though a little earlier may be appropriate for an older child who is over four. Don't worry about the techniques or whether your child uses oil. You can show him a couple of simple things (like the Open Book stroke on the chest or the I Love You stroke on the tummy) and then let him do it as he pleases. He will at first be hesitant and may need your encouragement to touch the baby. He might stroke her only a few times. But even the tiniest amount of contact will be very beneficial. Be sure to express your pleasure and pride to your child. Let him know that he did a good job and that his massaging is valuable to the baby.

Healthy Touch

Parents are concerned about the touching their children receive, and about helping them protect themselves from unhealthy individuals who may take advantage of them. Unfortunately, because of the fear engendered by media stories of molested children, many parents are giving their children frightening, negative messages about touch.

It is important that our children know the difference between healthy and unhealthy touching. Infant massage is a way to positively teach a child the difference. A child who has been massaged from infancy has several advantages over the child who is simply educated or warned about unhealthy or unwanted touch. The massaged child knows what healthy, loving touch feels like. Because of the emotional bonds it produces between parent and child, he feels close to his parents and tends to talk about his feelings more often. Thus he will be much more likely to report to his parents if he is concerned about the way someone talked to him or tried to touch him. In addition, massage time becomes "talking time," a time when parent and child can discuss things that are important to both of them. It is a perfect opportunity to talk about touching with your older child, and to help him learn how to protect himself. You can tell him, "Always tell me or Daddy or your teacher if somebody tries to touch you in a way that you don't like. I promise, no matter what, you will be safe." The type of interaction afforded by regular massage and Touch Relaxation helps your child develop a positive self-image and a sense of ownership of his body. He also develops a keen awareness of feelings and body language. The respect we show in asking permission to massage and to move to different parts of the body teaches him that people should ask his permission for intimate touch.

In general, massaged children grow up feeling confident and comfortable in their bodies, and they openly communicate with their parents. It is a tradition with long-term benefits, and it is definitely worth the effort!

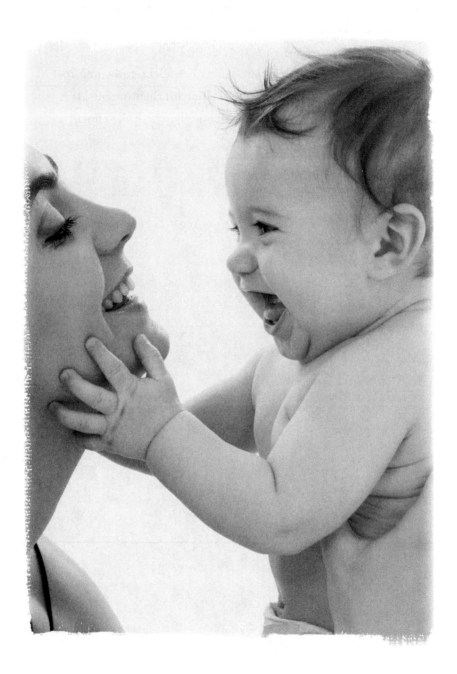

Chapter 19

Your Adopted or Foster Children

Not flesh of my flesh
Nor bone of my bone
But still miraculously my own.
Never forget for a single minute
You didn't grow under my heart,
But in it.

—ANONYMOUS

Attachment

Adoptive and foster parents are some of the most loving parents in the world. They choose their children, often children with medical problems and/or impairments, or children from races and cultures other than their own. These parents have a great deal of love to give. Yet it is common for their babies and children to resist affection.

Some past bonding theories have suggested that true bonding may not be possible between parents and children who are adopted or fostered. But simple evidence now proves that adoptive and foster parents can bond and form the same kinds of attachments that biological parents and their children form. Researchers David Brodinsky, Leslie Singer, Mary Stein, and Douglas Ramsey, among others, have found no difference in the development of parents' attachment to adopted and biological babies of the same age. If adoptive or foster parents provide a familial atmosphere—a warm, affectionate, and consistent response to a baby's needs—trust is learned and an attachment develops.

Lois Melina, an expert on adoption issues, cautions adoptive parents not to be too eager and overwhelm their new baby with affection. Often babies who come from a foster home or an orphanage are resistant to touch and affection, as well as easily overwhelmed by it. In addition, they must grieve the loss of their previous caregivers and homes and be allowed to gradually become part of their new family and environment. Gail Steinberg, of the online group Pact, An Adoption Alliance, and the author of *Bonding and Attachment: How Does Adoption Affect a Newborn?* says, "The best signals for knowing you're on track will come from the baby. Gather strength from simple pleasures: smiles and developmental milestones are proud signs of growth. Baby may take more or less time to attach than you do. Your partner may take more or less time. It may take days, weeks, months, or a year. Don't feel like a failure if attachment takes longer than you imagined. Most important is building a family together, no matter how long it takes."

Entire articles have been written about what's been called post-adoption depression syndrome. Often adoptive parents go through months and even years of what author June Bond calls "infertility hell," then go through an often prolonged adoption process. After the wonderful first days or weeks of having your new baby at home, it is not uncommon for one or both parents to experience feelings of anxiety, inadequacy, confusion, and a kind of letdown blues. Often when we reach a long-held goal, we experience anticlimax—the natural loss of the high arousal felt on the way to reaching a goal. You may also contend with feelings of guilt for the birth mother's grief and loss, stress from the expense, and perhaps dismay at discovering previously unknown or undisclosed health problems and background information about your child. Often adopted babies have attachment disorders, difficult adjustment periods, and overwhelming needs. Just like a biological parent, you may go through emotional ups and downs, lack of sleep, increased responsibilities, and higher stress levels. Joining an adoptive parents' support group helps some parents feel validated, as others in the group share your concerns. People further down the road can help you see that these feelings change, recognize developmental milestones, and avoid the difficulties that many first-time parents experience.

The new baby will experience both the normal stresses and the added stress of adjusting to a new environment, new caregivers, new sights, sounds, smells, tastes, and rhythms. Sometimes a newly adopted baby regresses for a time, withdraws from touch, and eventually cries deeply and uncontrollably. Read Chapter 14 again and use all your listening skills to help your baby grieve and cry in the safety of your love. Often babies won't begin to fuss and cry until they feel safe to do so—you can consider it a positive milestone when your baby or child begins to express her grief, anger, or even rage around you. Remember this as your baby grows older, for these feelings can surface again and again, and the best thing you can do is listen, allow venting to occur, and let your child know she is loved without condition.

Making Transitions

Try to find out as much as you can about the baby's previous environment and caregiving routine, who took care of her, what her birth was like, what formulas or foods she was given, and what colors, sounds, and smells she is accustomed to. Try to replicate some of these to allow her the comfort of the old while adapting to the new. For example, adoption expert Anna Marie Merrill suggests the following, which I hope will spark ideas about how to create a transitional environment for your baby:

- If a foster mother or previous caregiver used a certain perfume or scent, put a dab on a hanky for the baby's crib or rest place.
- If the baby is accustomed to a propped bottle, prop her bottle, but hold her while she is being fed.

- Begin eye contact by playing peekaboo and other eye contact games that give the baby a chance to make brief eye contact, feel its safety, and gradually move to more extended interaction.
- If the baby is used to being swaddled, use swaddling at home to help him bring his energies to center after a period of grief-release crying.
- For older babies, put food (such as Cheerios) into her mouth with your fingers instead of having her pick them up. This allows a little skin-to-skin contact, building trust.
- If the baby seems to withdraw from touch, try the Resting Hands technique for a while before trying massage. When you do begin the massage, emphasize the permission period and carefully watch your baby's cues. Be sure you are deeply relaxed yourself, and focused softly on him. If even Resting Hands is too much, step back further, perhaps leaving the clothing on and holding his legs or feet for a very short period. Gradually work up from there as your baby's cues indicate he is ready for more.
- Learn about the music, songs, or sounds the baby may have been accustomed to hearing and feeling in her previous environment, and use them during short periods throughout the day.
- Many countries water down formula or add a lot of sugar to it. Though you may not agree with these practices, you can begin using the same formula, gradually increasing the substance and decreasing the sugar or water content. Be aware of lactose intolerance; many babies from less developed countries or who have been breastfed may react poorly to the rich cow's milk we drink in the West.
- Instead of those crisp, new baby clothes you'd love to dress your new child in, find some soft, well-worn used clothing. Try to find out about and obtain the same laundry soap that was used in the baby's previous environment. The clothing will then smell familiar to him. Cut labels from the back of the clothing, as these may feel scratchy and irritating.

· If your baby has come from an orphanage where all the walls were painted the same color, say a bright sky blue, you might consider painting her room the same color for a while.

These types of transitional changes can help the baby feel more open to his new surroundings and less fearful, with familiar sights and sounds to soothe him. Merrill agrees that it is important to allow adopted and foster babies time to grieve. Do not hush every fuss or cry, but rather talk to the baby, allowing him to cry out his frustrations, fears, anger, grief, pain, and loneliness. If children are not allowed to do this in infancy (and sometimes even when they are), they will often act out violently when they are older, when they know it is "safe enough to misbehave." They will test you to see if you still love them when they are not on their best behavior.

Your new baby may be able to handle only one or two sources of stimulation at a time, so don't overload her by singing, massaging, and having a television or radio or computer or phone in the background. Present one interaction at a time, such as eye contact or singing or massage, but do not combine them until she is ready.

Gail Steinberg suggests continuing to show affection to your new baby, even though he may arch, stiffen, and seem to reject it. But don't force him. If eye contact is threatening, try small doses from a distance, and allow your baby to watch you when you change his clothing, feed, and bathe him without necessarily looking back. Allow him to gradually develop comfort with closeness.

One story, told to me by Anna Marie Merrill, demonstrates beautifully how one creative mother used this gradual process to achieve closeness with her adopted older son. She made a game wherein she would hold one end of a scarf, the boy the other. She would pull the scarf toward her a tiny bit, and then wait until he did so, too. It took a long time, but eventually their hands met, and the safety of attachment had been achieved. Another mother used story time as a way to introduce her child to touch in a noninvasive and nonthreatening way. Each day at a certain time, she

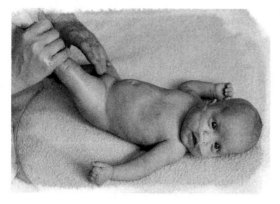

read the child a story as they sat in a rocking chair. Because the focus was on the story, the child could accept the physical contact.

Sometimes an adoptive or foster baby becomes attached to one parent but rejects the other. In this case, it is important for the rejected parent to find very gentle, slow methods to create the safety necessary for attachment. Merrill suggests that "nurturing dependence" is the beginning of creating attachment. Good things for the rejected parent to do would be to change, feed, or bathe the baby, if the baby can accept it. If not, give the baby some time and try again. Trust builds over time, and your consistent, accepting presence will foster the beginning of attachment cues to which you can respond.

Massaging the Adopted or Fostered Baby

Massaging an adopted or fostered baby is needed but can also be very difficult. Adoption expert Renee Henning says, "I do not want to overstate the difference between a baby from foster care or an orphanage and the average baby. There may be no difference in numerous cases. However, many babies from foster homes or orphanages do need good touching more than the average baby. Yet some of these babies may be initially less receptive to massage or less able to enjoy an extended massage than the average baby."

My suggestion is that you begin very slowly, using Resting Hands, with the baby fully clothed, and gradually move toward the entire massage presented in this book. Remember that your baby needs to grieve, and your best response is to validate her feelings and continue to offer loving touch, backing up when you need to, then moving forward again as trust and attachment grow. Nancy Verrier, in *Coming Home to Self: Healing the*

Primal Wound, says: "Children are creatures of sensation and intuition, and they know whether or not there is permission for them to experience and/or express their feelings." She stresses the importance of allowing your new baby to cry and feel understood. Often massage can help the baby begin to release these pent-up feelings of grief and fear.

Adoption expert Marlou Russell emphasizes the importance of finding this release. "Since loss is such a major part of adoption, grieving is a necessary and important process," she says. "Adoption can create a situation in which grieving is delayed or denied. Because adoption has been seen as such a positive solution, it may be difficult to feel that it is okay to grieve." This grief, when allowed—even encouraged—in infancy can help diminish later behavioral problems stemming from unresolved emotional pain. According to Leah LaGoy, another of Pact's online authors on adoption issues, the teenage years can restimulate the grief suppressed in babyhood because adolescence is a time of major transition and identity crisis. Teenagers often become angry at their adoptive parents; at least some of this is repressed rage at the birth parents, who they may unconsciously or consciously feel abandoned them.

If your adopted or foster baby responds negatively to your affectionate overtures, she may have some attachment or bonding disorder that can and should be addressed as soon as possible. The baby may not have received the response she needed in her previous environment, and she may have given up trying to get her needs met. When affection and responsiveness are finally offered, she may very likely react with stiffening, refusal to be consoled, and irritability. Don't take these behaviors personally. Validate the baby's feelings, and find ways to continue offering her loving touch and affection until she feels safe enough to relax into your love and accept your nurturing, including massage. All experts on attachment disorders stress the importance of addressing these issues as early in the baby's life as possible to prevent problems from surfacing later, be they social problems at school or pathological, sociopathic behavior. The older a child becomes, the more difficult it is to "rewire" the brain so as to be able to create and sustain healthy, interdependent, and loving relationships.

When teaching infant massage to foster parents, I was often asked, "Should I really massage this baby and help him resolve his grief, when he may be sent back into an abusive or neglectful situation?" My response is a resounding yes. Releasing his grief and fear, and accepting and experiencing healthy affection and attachment can help the baby be more resilient, healthier, and more independent. If he is sent back to abusive caregivers, his behavior with them may be different, causing a different response from them. For example, he may be more relaxed, smile more, be more "cuddly," and initiate eye contact more often. These behaviors can influence the caregivers to feel more loving and responsive toward him, thus changing their relationship and building more trust. If the caregivers can be taught good parenting skills and healthy, correct infant massage, so much the better.

As Terry Levy and Michael Orlans conclude, "The studies on attachment patterns, development and psychosocial functioning consistently show that children classified as securely attached in infancy do better in every important area of life as they develop." They show that these children solve problems more competently, are more resilient, make better friends, have higher self-esteem, are more independent, and receive more positive feedback from their environment.

Massaging your baby, whether you are an adoptive or a foster parent, can be one of the best things you can do for both yourself and your child to create loving, relaxed, open, healthy bonds that will stay with your baby for his or her entire life. What an incredible gift you can give: a legacy that can change the interactions of generations to come.

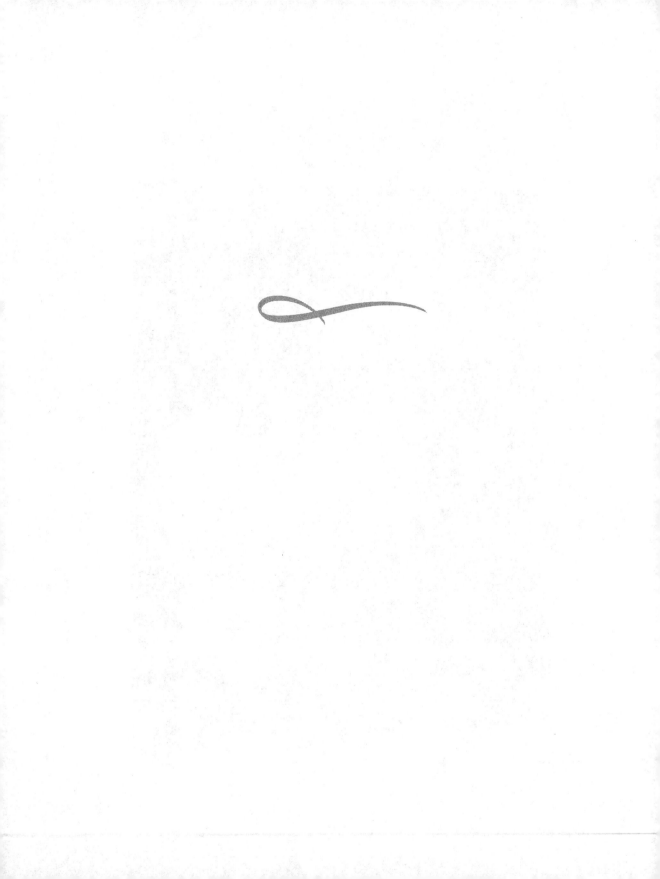

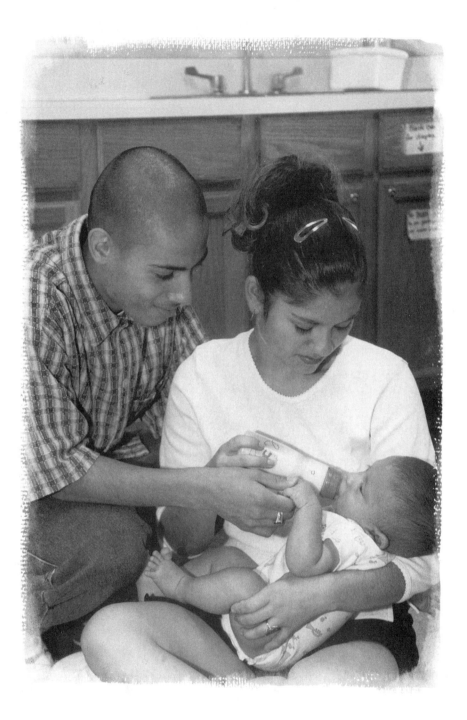

Chapter 20

A Note to Teen Parents

The best mothering
looks like no mothering.

Smothering heats up,
Stillness cools.
Be a still, cool stream
for your child's agitation.

A serene mother rocks
the universe in her arms,
and all is well.

—VIMALA MCCLURE,
THE TAO OF MOTHERHOOD

Massage and Bond with Your Baby

If you have decided to keep and raise your baby, you have made a very difficult choice, not only for yourself but for many of your loved ones, including your baby. If you have made that choice, I respect it, and I hope you have adults in your life who respect your choices and will support and help you. It is of utmost importance to both your future and that of your baby that you gather as much loving support and help from adults as you can. Don't let someone discourage you—just move on and keep searching out those people who can make up your little "village," for in this case it truly does take a village to raise a child. You will find yourself trying to navigate some pretty complicated waters. The decisions you will have to make will seem endless at times. Your body is constantly changing, and discomforts you never expected can make you irritable. Everyone has an opinion or advice to offer, some more destructive than constructive.

Whatever people say, you have made a choice, consciously or not, to become an adult before your biological programming or the culture may be ready for it. Stresses of education, family, relationships, physical discomforts, body image concerns, self-esteem, friendships, and medical issues can seem to bear down on you all at once. I won't try here to cover all of the issues you are dealing with. What I want to do is stress that your love for your baby has to become your number-one priority, and whatever supports that should be kept close and healthy. Whatever doesn't, put on the back burner or remove from your life—for the time being.

I encourage you to get good prenatal care, listen to your doctors, and read as much as you can about every aspect of this new phase of your life. Your baby's life and health—and yours—may depend on it. Take control of your life and with calm determination create a warm, safe, and loving environment into which you bring your baby and nourish your own spirit. If your mother isn't available, seek out the best mother you can think of and have the courage to ask her to help you be a good parent, even if it's only with occasional hugs, a listening heart, and answers to baby-care questions on the phone.

Massage is a great way to learn who your baby is and to begin the biological process that will create a loving and unbreakable bond between you. Even if you can't do it every day, try to find some way to work it in as a weekly or every-other-day ritual after your baby is born. Take an infant massage class from a Certified Infant Massage Instructor with IAIM if you can find one.

Remember the elements of the bonding process (Chapter 6), and try to get them all covered every day:

- Have skin-to-skin contact with your baby.
- Make warm and loving eye contact.
- Talk and play with your baby.
- Look at your baby's face when nursing or feeding him.
- Carry the baby on your chest for a little while each day.
- Avoid strong perfumes or scents the first three months.

Other important things to remember in those sleep-deprived months of early parenting:

- Never leave the baby alone or with people who you know are unreliable or uneducated in baby care.
- Never punish a baby either verbally or physically, and never use profanity in talking about or to your baby. If you feel stressed out and need some time to yourself, try to find someone to watch her for a little while. Fifteen minutes for a walk or deep breathing, or even dancing to your favorite music, can help get you in a better mood.
- Remember that crying is just a baby's way of talking, and babies sometimes have a lot to talk about. Never isolate the baby or punish her for crying.

Other things you can do are covered in this book, particularly the chapters about crying and fussing, colic, and attachment. What you do in the first year or two will lay a foundation for an entire lifetime. For teens, a year or two often seems like a long time, and I won't kid you—sometimes it's really hard and demands a lot more sacrifice than you thought. But hang in there. This is happening in your life for a reason, and later on you will be so glad and proud of yourself for being a good parent when it really counted. Beginning this way, you will find strengths you never knew you had. Your child will look to you to know how to be a good person, and being your child's role model will become an education in itself as you seek out the knowledge you need and continually improve yourself so your child will look to you with pride.

For Teen Fathers

As you already know, it takes more than making a baby to father a child. If you are having a baby, I encourage you to stay as close as possible to your baby. Even if you and the baby's mother are not together anymore, you can cooperate in coparenting. Try to make the environment as stress-free as possible for the baby's mother. Gather strength from any adult male role model you can find: your own father, a counselor or coach at school, or a counselor from your local social services agency. Read some of the books suggested in "References and Recommendations," and take an active part in the entire process as much as you are able. You will be required to sacrifice a lot of what you may want for yourself in order to provide financial support for your family and bond with your baby.

If the baby's mother is punitive or uncooperative, do whatever it takes, including cooperating in coparenting counseling sessions together. Take whatever classes or workshops may be offered to you. Show the baby's mother that you are making your best effort to support your child both financially and emotionally. Being an active, everyday part of your baby's life will be one of the most important things you do in your life, one that you will look back upon with no regrets when you are older. If the baby's mother decides to put the baby up for adoption, many states now have open adoptions, and you can find out how best to be involved as the baby's biological father.

A solid, loving relationship with your child will enable both you and your child to succeed and be happy in the future. The joy you get from your child's love is worth every effort you make to be a good, solid, loving, responsible father and role model.

We are all realizing that the physical, emotional, mental, and spiritual well-being of our babies must come first and foremost, and we must be willing to sacrifice at the proper time, to step forward at the proper time, and never to abandon our children, regardless of the final outcome. It is a lot to ask, but you can do it if you make up your mind that it is what you want and need, both for yourself and for your baby.

Resources

International Association of Infant Massage—IAIM

IAIM International Website: iaim.net
Note: We have more than fifty Instructor Trainers all over the world.
    To find one, go to the IAIM International Website.

IAIM International Office:
Sylvia Lindgren
Heidenstams Gata 9
SE-422 47 Hisings Backa
Sweden
Email: info@iaim.net
Tel: +46 (0)31-528980
Mob: +46 (0)702566693

United States Chapter Website: infantmassageusa.org
Looking for an IAIM Certified Instructor in the United States
    (CIMI)? Go to the United States chapter website.

United States Office:
Infant Massage USA
34760 Center Ridge Rd. #39006
North Ridgeville, OH 44039
Tel: 1-800-497-5996

Looking for an IAIM Certified Instructor (CIMI) in another country? Go to the chapter website for your country. Otherwise, contact an Instructor Trainer through the international website or write or call the international office.

Founder: Vimala McClure
Email: vimalaji@comcast.net
Blogs: vimalaji.wordpress.com and IAIM International
    Newsletter: iaim.net
About Me: about.me/vimalamcclure

For chapters of IAIM outside the United States, please contact the international office. We are growing quickly all over the world, and there will be many more instructors, trainers, and websites as the years pass. Most chapters and instructor trainers have websites, email addresses, phone or fax numbers, and you can find them through the international website.

A word of caution: Just because someone is a massage therapist does not mean they know how to teach infant massage. Be cautious about programs offered online. Some massage therapists think they can make up a series of strokes and then teach them as infant massage. But infant massage is not at all like adult massage, and it is not a "playtime" or "gymnastic" exercise. To properly teach infant massage, someone must know not only how a baby's body works but also the significance of the relationship between the caregiver and the baby, the way the baby's responses change as he or she grows, what a baby's cues mean, and many other subtle aspects of parent-infant communication. Babies do not respond well to poking, tickling, deep tissue work, or massage that is too tentative and light.

Special babies with special needs also need a special way of being massaged. All babies must be followed in their growth periods and responded to with respect, genuineness, and above all, love. The infant massage we teach is based on the idea that massage is one of the best tools we have to continue the attachment process, and so how we massage the baby, the way the strokes are done and in what order, is very important.

The massage we teach is based on infant massage that is thousands of years old, proven in the laboratory of human experience. The routine I developed is based on age-old practices, put together in a way that works today. Each stroke (and the order of the strokes) is there for a reason. I named and organized the strokes to be of greatest benefit to most babies. I created the Colic Relief Routine, Touch Relaxation, Resting Hands, the concept of asking permission, and many other aspects of what is in this book. Of course, as you get to know your baby and learn the program, you will find your own way of massaging your baby that is just right for you. I believe it is important before improvising to first get the instruction properly from this book and/or an IAIM certified instructor. In this way, your improvisations will benefit and not ever harm your little one.

The many thousands of parents who have received our instruction since 1976 would echo these cautions. Most say they never realized how profound the experience was until they had read this book and/or finished a class series. Where your baby is concerned, nothing but the best should be your guide.

For people who are interested in becoming instructors, know that the IAIM is the gold standard for infant massage instruction. After years of comparing our program to others that are offshoots or invented programs, people tell us that our program is the best, most comprehensive instruction, and that this book is the first, best, and most comprehensive book on the subject.

Since I wrote the first edition of this book in 1979, infant massage has spread around the world. There are infant massage instructors teaching families in more countries around the world in such diverse areas as China, Croatia, Czech Republic, Finland, Indonesia, Namibia, Oman, Qatar, Russia, Saudi Arabia, Slovakia, Tchad, Vietnam, and Zimbabwe.

Early Head Start programs in the United States are using infant massage to help the families they support to become closer to their babies and understand their communication. An instructor says, "Infant massage is the most satisfying work I have ever done. One of the Early Head Start staff people I consult with told me: 'It is the most perfect thing to accomplish all our goals. It does everything we are hoping for.' Infant massage gets people to focus on what's going on with their baby. All the talk, all the hours we spend with families, yet infant massage just does it so quickly."

Physical and occupational therapists who work directly doing early intervention with families of children with special needs find that teaching the families to massage their babies both supports the families and directly aids the therapists in their work with their children. Infant massage helps parents learn supportive positioning for their babies. It helps families time their daily care of their infant by reading, interpreting, and responding to their baby's cues. For babies, massage supports their developing nervous systems and helps them self-regulate, along with aiding in digestive issues such as reflux and colic.

The director of a program for infants and their families says, "Teaching families how to massage and nurture their babies helps us achieve our program's goals of enhancing parent-infant interaction and promoting healthy growth and development. We saw immediate results with the improvement of bonding and parent-child interaction."

Day care providers teach families to massage their babies in the evenings and over the weekend, to help them reconnect with their baby and remain the most important influence in their child's life. Child life specialists and nurses working with families of hospitalized children find that infant massage can be used to engage parents in their child's care and prepare them for their return home. While hospitalized premature babies may not yet be ready for massage, Inga Warren, M.Sc., a consultant occupational therapist in neonatology and early intervention and a NIDCAP trainer at the Winnicott Baby Unit in London, says:

"Reading the baby," the art of tuning into a baby's behavioral cues, is a significant component of the IAIM approach. The dialogue between the baby and parent, an important influence on every child's development, needs particularly fine tuning in the case of

preterm infants whose sensitivity to stimulation makes them highly vulnerable, easily overwhelmed and difficult to read.

Massaging delicate babies in the neonatal unit can easily be such an overwhelming experience and understanding the link between touch and communication is an essential part of safely guiding parents and babies towards confident, loving contact. As a developmental specialist on a neonatal intensive care unit that employs an IAIM trained nurse, I see this approach as a valuable contribution to an individualized developmental program that sees the baby as an active agent determining how we respond. Listening to the baby and the parents comes first, and this makes the IAIM way amenable for very small babies who may not be ready for massage at all but who will benefit, now and in the future, from the power of comforting parental touch.

Classes in infant massage are offered as parent education in many hospitals. One nurse told us, "Infant massage has really given me a new tool to be excited about and has really enriched our parent education program at the hospital. I had one mom of a three-month-old tell me that her daughter slept for seven hours straight for the first time after infant massage class. She was amazed!"

Social workers find that infant massage is a wonderful way to help parents form a deep connection with their child. A social worker in the United States shared: "I watched the fathers and babies light up; it was as if I could physically see the bond that connects them. It really felt good for me to see such immediate results with all the families who participated in the five-week course. In the work I do as a social worker I don't usually see immediate improvement in working with children and families. It was very heartwarming work, and seeing and hearing family members get closer to one another through infant massage was very powerful." Research has shown that infant massage can also be a tool to help reduce postnatal depression.

References and Recommendations

You will notice many of these studies are very old. That is because often they were the first groundbreaking studies and have since been proven over and over again. I feel the first studies are the most important, and they are the ones from which I drew my conclusions many years ago, so I do not list here every study that has been done on these subjects since then. In addition, in a book such as this one, footnotes are distracting. Therefore, the studies I refer to in the text are listed by chapter (but not specifically by page or line) and in alphabetical order, to make it easier for you to look them up yourself. Following are each chapter's references as well as books, video, and music I recommend to parents; not every chapter has recommended books.

Chapter 1: Why Massage Your Baby?

References

Adamson, S. "Hands-on Therapy." *Health Visitor* 66:2 (February 1993).

———. "Teaching Baby Massage to New Parents." *Complementary Therapies in Nursing and Midwifery* 2:6 (December 1996).

Ainsworth, M. *Infancy in Uganda: Infant Care and the Growth of Love.* Baltimore: Johns Hopkins University Press, 1967.

Auckett, A. "Baby Massage: An Alternative to Drugs." *Australian Nurses Journal* 9:5 (November 1979).

Barnard, K. E., and T. B. Brazelton, eds. *Touch: The Foundation of Experience.* Madison, WI: International University Press, 1990.

Brown, C., et al., eds. *The Many Facets of Touch.* Johnson & Johnson Pediatric Round Table, no. 10. New York: Elsevier, 1984.

Carpenter, E. *Eskimo Realities.* New York: Holt, Rinehart & Winston, 1973.

Curran, F. "Massage: A skill at our fingertips." *Modern Midwife,* July 1996.

Day, L. "Infant Massage." *Massage Magazine* 1:5 (1986).

Dellinger-Bavolek, J. "Infant massage: Communicating love through touch." *International Journal of Childbirth Education* 11:4 (December 1996).

Devore, I., et al. *Ethology and Psychiatry.* Toronto: University of Toronto Press, 1974.

Field, T. "Infant massage." *Zero to Three* 14:2 (1993).

———. "Infant massage." *Journal of Perinatal Education* 3:3 (1994).

———. "Massage therapy for infants and children." *Journal of Developmental and Behavioral Pediatrics* 16:2 (April 1995).

Goleman, D. "Pattern of love charted in studies." *New York Times,* September 10, 1985.

Isherwood, D. "Baby massage groups." *Modern Midwife,* February 1994.

Kaur, J. *Cuddles of Love: Nurturing Your Child with Loving Touch.* Singapore: MPH Group Publishing, 2015.

McClure (Schneider), V. "Infant massage." *Childbirth Educator* 5:4 (Summer 1986).

Pearce, J. *Magical Child.* New York: Dutton, 1977.

Plotsker-Herman, C. "The gentle art of infant massage." *American Baby Magazine,* March 1986.

Queen, S., and R. Habenstein. *The Family in Various Cultures.* New York: Lippincott, 1961.

Schneider, E. F. "The power of touch: Massage for infants." *Massage Magazine* 28 (1990).

Sullivan, L. E. "The gift of touch." *American Baby Magazine,* August 1995.

Trotter, R. "The play's the thing: Baby massage." *Psychology Today,* January 1987.

Zborowski, M., and E. Herzog. *Life Is with People.* New York: International Universities Press, 1952.

Recommended Books

Baldwin, R. *Special Delivery.* Berkeley, CA: Celestial Arts, 1995.

Berends, P. B. *Whole Child, Whole Parent.* New York: Harper, 1997.

Eisenberg, A., H. Murkoff, and S. Hathaway. *What to Expect the First Year.* New York: Workman Publishing, 2014.

Kaur, J. *Cuddles of Love: Nurturing Your Child with Loving Touch.* Singapore: MPH Group Publishing, 2015.

Leach, P. *Babyhood.* New York: Alfred A. Knopf, 1989.

Leboyer, F. *Loving Hands: The Traditional Art of Baby Massage.* New York: Newmarket, 1997.

Maiden, A. H., and E. Farwell. *The Tibetan Art of Parenting: From Before Conception Through Early Childhood.* Boston: Wisdom Publications, 2008.

Sears, M., and W. Sears. *25 Things Every New Mother Should Know.* Boston: Harvard Common Press, 2009.

———. *The Baby Book: Everything You Need to Know About Your Baby from Birth to Age Two.* Boston: Little, Brown, 2003.

Stillerman, E. *Mother Massage: A Handbook for Relieving the Discomforts of Pregnancy.* New York: Dell, 2006.

Chapter 2: Your Baby's Sensory World

References

Bernhardt, J. "Sensory capabilities of the fetus." *Maternal Child Nursing* 12 (January-February 1987).

Birnholtz, J. "The development of human fetal eye movement patterns." *Science* 213 (August 7, 1981).

Bower, T. "The visual world of infants." *Scientific American* 215 (December 1966).

Condon, W., and L. W. Sander. "Neonate movement is synchronized with adult speech: Interactional participation and language acquisition." *Science* 183 (June 1974).

Day, S. "Mother-infant activities as providers of sensory stimulation." *American Journal of Occupational Therapy* 36:9 (December 1982).

DeCasper, A., et al. "Of human bonding: Newborns prefer their mother's voices." *Science* 208 (June 6, 1980).

Fantz, R. "Maturation of pattern vision in young infants." *Journal of Comparative and Physiological Psychology* 55 (1962).

———. "Pattern vision in newborn infants." *Science* 140 (1963).

Ferreira, A. "Emotional factors in the prenatal environment." *Journal of Nervous and Mental Diseases* 141 (1965).

Field, T., S. Schnaberg, F. Scaridi, C. Bauer, N. Vega-Lahr, R. Garcia, J. Nystrom, and C. Kuhn. "Tactile/kinesthetic stimulation effects on preterm neonates." *Pediatrics* 77 (May 1986).

———. "Touch for socioemotional and physical well-being: A review." *Developmental Review* 30:4 (2011): 367–83.

Figar, W. P., and C. Moon. "Psychology of newborn auditory preferences." *Seminars in Perinatology* 13 (1989).

Goleman, D. "The experience of touch: Research points to a critical role." *New York Times,* February 2, 1988.

Hooker, D. *The Prenatal Origins of Behavior.* Lawrence: University of Kansas Press, 1952.

Kaur, J. *Cuddles of Love: Nurturing Your Child with Loving Touch.* Singapore: MPH Group Publishing, 2015.

Kellen, A. "Babies understand 'baby talk,' research suggests." *CNN Interactive,* March 18, 1999.

Kuhl, P. K., et al., "Cross-language analysis of phonetic units in language addressed to infants," *Science* 5326 (August 1, 1997).

Liley, A. "The fetus as a personality." *Australian and New Zealand Journal of Psychiatry* 6 (1972).

Ludington-Hoe, S., and S. Golant. *How to Have a Smarter Baby*. New York: Rawson Associates, 1990.

McCarthy, P. "Scent: The tie that binds?" *Psychology Today,* July 1986.

Montagu, A. "The skin and human development." *Somatics* 1:3 (Fall 1977).

Murkoff, H., and S. Mazel. *What to Expect When You're Expecting,* 4th ed. New York: Workman Publishing, 2015.

Pederson, P., et al. "Evidence for olfactory function in utero." *Science* 221 (July 29, 1983).

Porter, R., et al. "The importance of odors in mother-infant interactions." *Maternal Child Nursing* 12 (Fall 1983).

Restak, R. *The Infant Mind*. New York: Doubleday, 1986.

Rowland, R. "Babies learn language lessons before they talk, study shows." *CNN Interactive,* December 31, 1998.

Spence, M., and A. De Caster. "Prenatal experience with low-frequency maternal voice sounds influences neonatal perception of maternal voice sales." *Infant Behavior and Development* 10 (1987).

Stack, D. "The Salience of Touch and Physical Contact During Infancy: Unraveling Some of the Mysteries of the Somesthetic Sense." Chapter 13 in *Blackwell Handbook of Infant Development,* 1994.

Valman, H., and T. Pearson. "What the fetus feels." *British Medical Journal* 280 (1980).

Verney, T., and T. Kelly. *The Secret Life of the Unborn Child: How You Can Prepare Your Baby for a Happy, Healthy Life*. New York: Dell, 1988.

Williams, H. Personal interview by author, 1987.

Chapter 3: The Importance of Skin Stimulation

References

Fitzgerald, H., et al. *Child Nurturance: Studies of Development in Non-human Primates,* vol. 3. New York: Putnam, 1982.

Harlow, H., and M. Harlow. "Learning to love." *American Scientist* 54 (1959).

———. "Effects of various mother-infant relationships on rhesus monkey behaviors." In *Determinants of Infant Behavior,* vol. 4, ed. B. M. Foss (London: Methuen, 1969).

Hunt, D. *Parents and Children in History*. New York: Basic Books, 1970.

Karen, R. *Becoming Attached: First Relationships and How They Shape Our Capacity to Love*. New York: Oxford University Press, 1998.

Kaur, J. *Cuddles of Love: Nurturing Your Child with Loving Touch*. Singapore: MPH Group Publishing, 2015.

Ottenbacher, K. J., et al. "The effectiveness of tactile stimulation as a form of early intervention: Quantitative evaluation." *Developmental and Behavioral Pediatrics* 8:2 (1987).

Prescott, J. "Pleasure/violence reciprocity theory: The distribution of 49 cultures, relating infant physical affection to adult physical violence." *Futurist,* April 1975.

Rheingold, H. *Maternal Behavior in Mammals.* New York: Van Nostrand Reinhold, 1963.

Rice, R. "Premature infants respond to sensory stimulation." *APA Monitor,* November 1975.

———. "Cardiac and behavioral responses to tactile stimulation in premature and full term infants." *Developmental Psychology* 12:4 (July 1976).

———. "Neurophysiological development in premature infants." *Developmental Psychology* 12:4 (July 1976).

———. "Neurophysiological development in premature infants following stimulation." *Developmental Psychology* 13 (1977).

Roberts, M. "Baby love." [Effects of infant experience on later adult love life, a study by Shaver and Hazan.] *Psychology Today,* March 1987.

Rorke, L., and H. Riggs. *Myelination of the Brain in the Newborn.* Philadelphia: Lippincott, 1969.

Slater, C. "The effects of tactile stimulation on infants." *Massage Magazine* 28 (1990).

Whittlestone, W. "The physiology of early attachment in mammals: Implications for human obstetric care." *Medical Journal of Australia* 1 (1978).

Yang, R., et al. "Newborn responses to threshold tactile stimulations," *Child Development* 45:1 (March 1974).

Chapter 4: Stress and Relaxation

References

Benson, H. *The Relaxation Response.* New York: Harper Collins, 2000.

———. *Beyond the Relaxation Response.* New York: Berkley Publishing Group, 1985.

Gooey, D. *The End of Stress: Four Steps to Rewire Your Brain.* New York: Atria, 2014.

Selye, H. *Stress Without Distress.* New York: New American Library, 1974.

Stott. "Children in the womb: Effects of stress." *New Society,* May 19, 1977.

Witkin-Lanoil, G. *The Female Stress Syndrome.* New York: Berkley Books, 1984.

Recommended Books

Benson, H. *The Relaxation Response.* New York: Harper Collins, 2000.

Selye, H. *Stress Without Distress.* New York: New American Library, 1974.

Stott. "Children in the womb: Effects of stress." *New Society,* May 19, 1977.

Witkin-Lanoil, G. *The Female Stress Syndrome.* New York: Berkley Books, 1984.

Chapter 5: Bonding, Attachment, and Infant Massage

References

Anisfeld, E., V. Casper, M. Noyce, and N. Cunningham. "Does infant carrying promote attachment? An experimental study of the effects of increased physical contact on the development of attachment." *Child Development* 61 (1990).

Caldwell, B. "The tie that binds: Does daycare weaken the bond with your baby?" *Working Mother,* April 1987.

Capra, F. *The Tao of Physics: An Exploration of the Parallels Between Modern Physics and Eastern Mysticism.* Boston: Shambhala Publications, 1999.

Courtney, J. *FirstPlay, Baby Massage, Story Telling: Four Weeks to Toddler.* Palm Beach Gardens, FL: Developmental Play & Attachment Therapies, 2015.

Curry, M. "Maternal attachment behavior and the mother's self-concept: The effect of early skin-to-skin contact." *Nursing Research* 31:2 (March-April 1982).

De Chateau, P., and B. Wiberg. "Long-term effect on mother-infant behavior of extra contact during the first hour postpartum." *Acta Pediatrica* 66 (1977).

D'Spagnat, B. "The quantum theory and reality." *Scientific American,* November 1979.

Edwards, C., et al. "The effects of daycare participation on parent-infant interaction at home." *American Journal of Orthopsychiatry* 57:1 (January 1987).

Hage, D. "Foundations of attachment." *International Concerns for Children,* 1999.

Karen, R. *Becoming Attached: First Relationships and How They Shape Our Capacity to Love.* New York: Oxford University Press, 1998.

Klaus, M., and J. Kennell. *Parent Infant Bonding.* St. Louis: Mosby, 1982.

———. *Bonding: The Beginning of Parent-Infant Attachment.* New York: New American Library, 1983.

Liedloff, J. *The Continuum Concept: In Search of Happiness Lost.* Reading, MA: Perseus, 2008.

Lorenz, K. *Evolution and the Modification of Behavior.* Chicago: University of Chicago Press, 1965.

Magid, K., and C. McKelvey. *High Risk: Children Without a Conscience.* New York: Bantam Books, 1987.

McKenna, J. J. *Babies Need Their Mothers Beside Them.* Natural Child Project Society, 1996.

Newton, R. *The Attachment Connection: Parenting a Secure and Confident Child Using the Science of Attachment Theory.* Oakland, CA: New Harbinger Publications, 2008.

Nicholson, B., and L. Parker. *Attached at the Heart: Eight Proven Parenting Principles for Raising Connected and Compassionate Children from Preconception to Age 5.* Deerfield Beach, FL: Health Communications 2013.

Pearce, J. *Magical Child.* New York: Penguin Books, 1977.

———. *Magical Child Matures.* New York: Penguin Books, 1978.

Prescott, J. "Pleasure/violence reciprocity theory: The distribution of 49 cultures, relating infant physical affection to adult physical violence." *Futurist,* April 1975.

Rader, L. *Attachment Parenting.* London: CICO Books, 2014.

Reite, M. "Touch, attachment, and health: Is there a relationship?" In *The Many Facets of Touch,* ed. C. Brown et al. Johnson & Johnson Pediatric Round Table, no. 10. New York: Elsevier, 1984.

Restak, R. *The Infant Mind.* New York: Doubleday, 1986.

Ringler, N., et al. "The effects of extra postpartum contact and maternal speech patterns on children's IQ, speech, and comprehension at five." *Child Development* 49 (1978).

Sears, W., and M. Sears. *The Attachment Parenting Book.* Cambridge, MA: Perseus, 1985.

Ziglar, E. "Recommendations of the Yale Bush Center Advisory Committee on Infant Care Leave." Hearing on Parental Leave HR 2020 Before House Subcommittees on Civil Service, Labor Management Relations, Labor Standards, and Employee Benefits (October 17, 1985). Washington, DC: U.S. Government Printing Office, 1985.

Recommended Books

Brazelton, T. B. *Earliest Relationships: Parents, Infants, and the Drama of Early Attachment.* Reading, MA: Perseus, 2012.

Brazelton, T. B., and J. Sparrow. *Touchpoints: Your Child's Emotional and Behavioral Development.* Reading, MA: Perseus, 2006.

Briggs, D. C. *Your Child's Self-Esteem.* New York: Broadway Books, 2001.

Granju, K., and B. Kennedy. *Attachment Parenting: Instinctive Care for Your Baby and Young Child.* New York: Pocket Books, 1999.

Karen, R. *Becoming Attached: First Relationships and How They Shape Our Capacity to Love.* New York: Oxford University Press, 1998.

Kaur, J. *Cuddles of Love: Nurturing Your Child with Loving Touch.* Singapore: MPH Group Publishing, 2015.

Klaus, M., J. Kennell, and P. Klaus. *Bonding: Building the Foundations of Secure Attachment and Independence.* Reading, MA; Perseus, 1996.

Leach, P. *Children First: What Society Must Do—and Is Not Doing—for Children Today.* New York: Random House, 2011.

Wiessinger, D., D. West, L. Smith, and T. Pitman. *Sweet Sleep: Nighttime and Naptime Strategies for the Breastfeeding Family.* New York: Ballantine Books, 2014.

Chapter 6: The Elements of Bonding

Austin, P. "Synchronous movements to human speech." *Perceptual Motor Skills* 79 (1983).

Belsky, J., and L. Steinberg. "The effects of day care: A critical review." *Child Development* 49 (1978).

Chamberlain, D., *The Mind of Your Newborn Baby*. Berkeley, CA: North Atlantic Books, 1998.

Clary, E., et al. "Socialization and situational influences on sustained altruism." *Child Development* 57 (1986).

Curry, M. "Maternal attachment behavior and the mother's self-concept: The effect of early skin-to-skin contact." *Nursing Research* 31:2 (March-April 1982).

De Casper, A., et al. "Of human bonding: Newborns prefer their mothers' voices." *Science* 208 (June 6, 1980).

De Chateau, P., and B. Wiberg. "Long-term effect on mother-infant behavior of extra contact during the first hour postpartum." *Acta Pediatrica* 66 (1977).

Divitto, B., et al. "Talking and sucking: Infant feeding behavior and parent stimulation." *Infant Behavior and Development* 6:2 (April 1983).

Fagot, B. I., and K. Kavanagh. "The prediction of antisocial behavior from avoidant attachment classifications." *Child Development* 61 (1990).

Field, T., L. Guy, and V. Umbel. "Infants' responses to mother's imitative behaviors." *Infant Mental Health Journal* 6:1 (1985).

Gordon, J., and M. Goodavage. *The Happy Parents' Guide to the Family Bed (and a Peaceful Night's Sleep)*. New York: St. Martin's Press, 2002.

Hunziker, U., and R. Barr. "Increased carrying reduces infant crying: A randomized control trial." *Pediatrics* 77 (May 1986).

Klaus, M., and J. Kennell. *Parent Infant Bonding*. St. Louis: Mosby, 1982.

———. *Bonding: The Beginning of Parent-Infant Attachment*. New York: New American Library, 1983.

Kuroda, Kumi. "From mice to humans, comfort is being carried by mom." *ScienceDaily* (April 2013).

McKenna, J. J. *Babies Need Their Mothers Beside Them*. Natural Child Project Society, 1996.

———. *Sleeping with Your Baby : A Parent's Guide to Cosleeping*. Washington, DC: Platypus Media, 2007.

Medoff, M. "The gentle benefits of baby massage." *East West Journal* 16:2 (February 1986).

Newman, R. S., M. L. Rowe, and R. N. Berstein, "Input and uptake at 7 months predicts toddler vocabulary: The role of child-directed speech and infant processing skills in language development." *Journal of Child Language* 43:5 (2016): 1158–73.

Peretz, I., and M. Corbeil. "Babies remain calm twice as long when listening to song compared to speech." *Child Health News*, University of Montreal, 2015.

Reite, M. "Touch, attachment, and health: Is there a relationship?" In *The Many Facets of Touch*, ed. C. Brown et al. Johnson & Johnson Pediatric Round Table, no. 10. New York: Elsevier, 1984.

Restak, R. *The Infant Mind*. New York: Doubleday, 1986.

Ringler, N., et al. "The effects of extra postpartum contact and maternal speech patterns on children's IQ, speech, and comprehension at five." *Child Development* 49 (1978).

Roberts, M. "Baby love." [Effects of infant experience on later adult love life, study by Shaver and Hazan.] *Psychology Today*, March 1987.

Ronald, A. "Newborn's gaze predicts future childhood behavior." *Scientific Reports*, June 26, 2015.

Snow, C. "The development of conversations between mothers and babies." *Journal of Child Language* 4 (1977).

Springer, S., and G. Deutch. *Left Brain, Right Brain: Perspectives from Cognitive Neuroscience*. New York: Freeman, 2001.

Thevenin, T. *The Family Bed*. Wayne, NJ: Avery, 2002.

Wiessinger, D., D. West, L. Smith, and T. Pitman. *Sweet Sleep: Nighttime and Naptime Strategies for the Breastfeeding Family*. New York: Ballantine Books, 2014.

Ziglar, E. "Recommendations of the Yale Bush Center Advisory Committee on Infant Care Leave." Hearing on Parental Leave HR 2020 Before House Subcommittees on Civil Service, Labor Management Relations, Labor Standards, and Employee Benefits (October 17, 1985). Washington, DC: U.S. Government Printing Office, 1985.

Recommended Books
See Chapter 5.

Chapter 7: Attachment and the Benefits of Infant Massage

Bowlby, J. *Attachment and Loss*. New York: Basic Books, 1996.

Condon, W., and L. Sander. "Neonate movement is synchronized with adult speech: Interactional participation and language acquisition." *Science* 183 (June 1974).

Crockenberg, S. "Infant irritability, mother responsiveness, and social support influences in the security of infant-mother attachment." *Child Development* 52 (1981).

Curry, M. "Maternal attachment behavior and the mother's self-concept: The effect of early skin-to-skin contact." *Nursing Research* 31:2 (March-April 1982).

Ehrlich, D. "The daddy diaries. Chapter 24. A Buddhist view of attachment parenting." *Huffington Post*, November 11, 2015.

Fagot, B. I., and K. Kavanagh. "The prediction of antisocial behavior from avoidant attachment classifications." *Child Development* 61 (1990).

Granju, K., and B. Kennedy. *Attachment Parenting: Instinctive Care for Your Baby and Young Child*. New York: Pocket Books, 1999.

Newton, R. *The Attachment Connection: Parenting a Secure and Confident Child Using the Science of Attachment Theory.* Oakland, CA: New Harbinger Publications, 2008.

Recommended Books
See Chapter 5.

Chapter 8: Especially for Fathers

References

Block, J. *Lives Through Time.* Berkeley, CA: Bancroft Books, 1971.

Daly, T. "Men, infant massage, and manhood." *Tender Loving Care* [newsletter of the International Association of Infant Massage], Winter 1987.

De Casper A., et al. "Human newborns' perception of male voices: Preference, discrimination, and reinforcing value." *Developmental Psychobiology* 17:5 (September 1984).

Giefer, M. A., and C. Nelson. "A method to help new fathers develop parenting skills." *Journal of Obstetric, Gynecologic, and Neonatal Nursing* 10:6 (November-December 1981).

Kennell, J., et al. *Parent Infant Bonding.* St. Louis: Mosby, 1982.

Lamb, M. *The Role of the Father in Child Development.* New York: Wiley, 1981.

Lozoff, M. "Fathers and autonomy in women." In *Women and Success,* ed. R. Kundsin. New York: Morrow, 1974.

Pannabacker, B., et al. "The effect of early extended contact on father-newborn interaction." *Journal of Genetic Psychology* 141 (September 1982).

Parke, R. "Father infant interaction." In *Maternal Attachment and Mothering Disorders.* Johnson & Johnson Pediatric Round Table. New York: Elsevier, 1978.

———. "Father-infant interaction and infant social responsiveness." In *The Handbook of Infant Development,* ed. J. Osofsky. New York: Wiley, 1979.

Taub, D., ed. *Primate Paternalism.* New York: Van Nostrand Reinhold, 1984.

Tuttman, S. "The father's role in the child's development of the capacity to cope with separation and loss." *Journal of the American Academy of Psychoanalysis,* July 1986.

Zaslow, M., et al. "Depressed mood in fathers: Associations with parent-infant interaction." *Genetic, Social, and General Psychology Monographs* 3:2 (May 1985).

Recommended Books

Brott, A. *The New Father: A Dad's Guide to the First Year.* New York: Abbeville Press, 2015.

DeMorier, E. *Crib Notes for the First Year of Fatherhood.* Minneapolis: Fairview Press, 1998.

Engledow, D. *Confessions of the World's Best Father*. New York: Penguin Group, 2014.

Harrison, H. *Father to Daughter: Life Lessons on Raising a Girl*. New York: Workman Publishing, 2013.

———. *Father to Son: Life Lessons on Raising a Boy*. New York: Workman Publishing, 2013.

Heinowitz, J. *Fathering Right from the Start: Straight Talk About Pregnancy, Birth, and Beyond*. Novato, CA: New World Library, 2001.

Jamiolkowski, R. *A Baby Doesn't Make the Man: Alternative Sources of Power and Manhood for Young Men*. Teen Pregnancy Prevention Library, 1997.

Karen, R. *Becoming Attached: First Relationships and How They Shape Our Capacity to Love*. New York: Oxford University Press, 1998.

Mactavish, S. *The New Dad's Survival Guide: Man-to-Man Advice for First-Time Fathers*. Boston: Little, Brown, 2005.

Marcello, J. *Fathers and Babies: How Babies Grow and What They Need from You, from Birth to Eighteen Months*. New York: HarperCollins, 1993.

Meeker, M. *Strong Fathers, Strong Daughters: 10 Secrets Every Father Should Know*. Brentwood, TN: A Group, 2012.

Meyer, D., ed. *Uncommon Fathers: Reflections on Raising a Child with a Disability*. Bethesda, MD: Woodbine House, 1995.

Miller, F., and S. J. Bacharach. *Cerebral Palsy: A Complete Guide for Caregiving*. Baltimore: Johns Hopkins University Press, 1995.

Murdock, M. *Uncommon Father: 31 Qualities of Every Successful Father*. Wisdom International, 2013.

Ogden, P. W. *The Silent Garden: Raising Your Deaf Child*. Washington, DC: Gallaudet University Press, 1982.

Parke, R., and A. Brott. *Throwaway Dads: The Myths and Barriers That Keep Men from Being the Fathers They Want to Be*. New York: Houghton Mifflin, 1999.

Payleitner, J. *52 Things Kids Need from a Dad: What Fathers Can Do to Make a Lifelong Difference*. Eugene, OR: Harvest House Publishers, 2010.

Rayburn, P. *Do Fathers Matter? What Science Is Telling Us About the Parent We've Overlooked*. New York: Farrar, Straus and Giroux, 2014.

Sears, W. *Becoming a Father*. Franklin Park, IL: La Leche League International, 2003.

Chapter 9: Helping Baby (and You) Learn to Relax

References

Benson, H. *The Relaxation Response*. New York: HarperCollins, 2000.

Davis, M., et al. *The Relaxation and Stress Reduction Workbook*. New York: New Harbinger, 2008.

Debelle, B. "Relaxation and Baby Massage." *Australian Nurses Journal* 10:5 (May 1981).

Diamond, A., A. Churchland, L. Cruess, and N. Z. Kirkham. "Early developments in the ability to understand the relation between stimulus and reward." *Developmental Psychology* 35 (1999): 1507–17.

Kabat-Zinn, J. *Full Catastrophe Living: Using the Wisdom of Your Body and Mind to Face Stress, Pain, and Illness.* New York: Bantam, 2015.

Schaper, K. "Towards a calm baby and relaxed parents." *Family Relations: Journal of Applied Family and Child Studies* 31:3 (July 1982).

Selye, H. *Stress Without Distress.* New York: New American Library, 1974.

Stahl, B., and E. Goldstein. *A Mindfulness-Based Stress Reduction Workbook.* [Includes web link to 21 guided meditations.] Oakland, CA: New Harbinger Publications, 2010.

Recommended Books

Benson, H. *The Relaxation Response.* New York: HarperCollins, 2000.

Benson, H., and W. Proctor. *Beyond the Relaxation Response: How to Harness the Healing Power of Your Personal Beliefs.* New York: Berkley, 1994.

Davis, M., et al. *The Relaxation and Stress Reduction Workbook.* New York: New Harbinger, 2008.

McClure, V. *A Woman's Guide to Tantra Yoga.* Novato, CA: New World Library, 1997.

———. *The Path of Parenting: Twelve Principles to Guide Your Journey.* Novato, CA: New World Library, 1999.

Chapter 10: Your Baby's Brain

References

Chamberlain, D. *The Mind of Your Newborn Baby.* Berkeley, CA: North Atlantic Books, 1998.

Courtney, J. *FirstPlay, Baby Massage, Story Telling: Ages Four Weeks to Toddler.* Developmental Play & Attachment Therapies, 2015.

Eliot, L. *What's Going On in There? How the Brain and Mind Develop in the First Five Years of Life.* New York: Bantam Books, 2000.

Epstein, H. "Phrenoblysis: Special brain and mind growth periods." In *Developmental Psychobiology.* New York: Wiley, 1974.

Gerhardt, S. *Why Love Matters: How Affection Shapes a Baby's Brain.* New York: Brunner- Routledge, 2004.

Hanson, R. *Buddha's Brain: The Practical Neuroscience of Happiness, Love, and Wisdom.* New York: New Harbinger Publications, 2009.

James, S. *Baby Brains: The Smartest Baby in the Whole World.* Cambridge, MA: Candlewick, 2007.

MacFarlane, Jo. "Mothers who experience stress or worry before pregnancy 'more likely to have babies who cry for longer.'" DailyMail.com.

Medina, J. *Brain Rules for Baby: How to Raise a Smart and Happy Child from Zero to Five*. Seattle, WA: Pear Press, 2014.

Reins, S., and J. Goldman. *The Development of the Brain*. Springfield, IL: Thomas, 1980.

Restak, R. *The Infant Mind*. New York: Doubleday, 1986.

Siegel, D., and T. Bryson. *The Whole-Brain Child: 12 Revolutionary Strategies to Nurture Your Child's Developing Mind*. New York: Bantam Books, 2011.

Recommended Books

Eliot, L. *What's Going On in There? How the Brain and Mind Develop in the First Five Years of Life*. New York: Bantam Books, 2000.

Legerstee, M., and D. Haley. *The Infant Mind: Origins of the Social Brain*. New York: Guilford Press, 2013.

Medina, J. *Brain Rules for Baby: How to Raise a Smart and Happy Child from Zero to Five*. Seattle, WA: Pear Press, 2014.

Restak, R. *The Infant Mind*. New York: Doubleday, 1986.

Siegel, D., and T. Bryson. *The Whole-Brain Child: 12 Revolutionary Strategies to Nurture Your Child's Developing Mind*. New York: Bantam Books, 2011.

Chapter 11: Music and Massage

References

Ayres, B. "Effects of infant carrying practices on rhythm in music." *Ethos* 1:4 (Winter 1973).

Bench, R. "Sound transmission to the human fetus through the maternal abdominal wall." *Journal of Genetic Psychology* 113–14 (1968–69).

Cass-Beggs, B. *Your Baby Needs Music*. New York: St. Martin's Press, 1978.

Daiken, L. *The Lullaby Book*. London: E. Ward, 1959.

Geestesleven, U. *Clump-a-Dump and Snickle-Snack: Pentatonic Songs for Children*. New York: Mercury Press, 1966.

Hill, D., S. Trehub, and K. Kamenetsky. "Mothers' and fathers' songs to infants." *Current Research in Music Cognition*, 1998.

Matterson, E. *This Little Puffin*. London: Penguin Books, 1972.

Opie, I., and P. Opie. *The Oxford Nursery Rhyme Book*. London: Oxford University Press, 1955.

Recommended Books

Andrews, J., and E. Hamilton. *Julie Andrews' Collection of Poems, Songs, and Lullabies*. [Includes exclusive CD.] Boston: Little, Brown, 2009.

Beall, P., and S. Hagen. *Wee Sing Nursery Rhymes and Lullabies*. New York: Putnam Books, 2002.

Chorao, K. *The Baby's Bedtime Book*. New York: E. P. Dutton, 1984.

Dyer, J. *Animal Crackers: A Delectable Collection of Pictures, Poems, and Lullabies for the Very Young.* Boston: Little, Brown, 1996.

Emerson, S., C. MacLean, and M. MacLean. *The Nursery Treasury: A Collection of Baby Games, Rhymes and Lullabies.* New York: Doubleday, 1988.

Feierabend, J. *The Book of Lullabies: Wonderful Songs and Rhymes Passed Down from Generation to Generation for Infants and Toddlers.* Chicago: GIA Publications, 2000.

Kapp, R. *Lullabies: An Illustrated Songbook.* New York: Harcourt Brace, 1997.

McKellar, S. *A Child's Book of Lullabies.* New York: DK Publishing, 1997.

Recommended Music

"Ami Tomake Bhalobashi Baby: The Bengali Lullaby," signature of the International Association of Infant Massage. Several different CDs available; infantmassagewarehouse.com.

Andrews, J., and E. Hamilton. *Julie Andrews' Collection of Poems, Songs, and Lullabies.* [Includes exclusive CD.] Boston: Little, Brown, 2009.

Authentic Cajun Lullabies. Mardi Gras CD.

Baby Genius. *Sweet Dream Lullabies.* IMT Corporation CD.

Beijing Angelic Choir. *Chinese Lullabies.* Wind CD.

Burell, T. *Sweet Baby Lullabies to Soothe Your Newborn.* CD.

Celtic Twilight 3: Lullabies. Hearts of Space CD.

Children's Songs from Around the World, Vol. 3: Lullabies—Asia, Latin America, Africa, Oceania. Arion CD.

DelRay, M. *Lullabies of Latin America.* WEA/Atlantic/Rhino CD.

Folk Music in Sweden, Vol. 6: Rhymes and Lullabies. Caprice CD.

Hawaii and Its Lullabies, Vol. 20. ANS Records CD.

Luck, S. "Ami Tomake Lullaby." 2 CDs. amitomake.com.

Lullabies for Little Angels: Sing Along. Madacy Records CD.

Lullabies: Growing Minds with Music. Twin Sisters Audio CD.

N'dege Ocello, M. *Plantation Lullabies.* WEA/Warner Bros. CD.

Palmer, H. *A Child's World of Lullabies.* Hap-Pal Music CD.

Re-Bops, The. *Daddy's Lullabies.* Rebop CD.

Yiddish Lullabies. Israel Music CD.

Chapter 12: Getting Ready

References

"At what temperature should you keep a baby?" [Editorial.] *Lancet* 2:1 (September 12, 1970).

Daga, S. R., L. Chandrashekhar, P. P. Pol, and S. Patole. "Appropriate technology in keeping babies warm in India." *Annals of Tropical Paediatrics,* March 1986.

Davis, A. *Let's Have Healthy Children.* New York: Harcourt Brace Jovanovich, 1972.

Glas, N. *Conception, Birth, and Early Childhood*. Spring Valley, NY: Anthroposophic Press, 1972.

Johanson, R. B., S. A. Spencer, P. Rolfe, P. Jones, and D. S. Massa. "Effect of post-delivery care on neonatal body temperature." *Acta Pediatrica* 81:11 (November 1992).

Rutter, N. "Response of term babies to a warm environment." *Archives of the Disabled Child* 53 (March 1979).

Strothers, J., et al. "Thermal balance and sleep state in the newborn infant in a cool environment." *Journal of Physiology* 273 (December 1977).

Wolff, P. "The causes, controls, and organization of behavior in the neonate." *Psychological Issues* [Monograph 17] 5 (1965).

Chapter 13: How to Massage Your Baby

References

Berkson, D. *The Foot Book: Healing with the Integrated Treatment of Foot Reflexology*. New York: Funk & Wagnalls, 1977.

Crelin, E. *Functional Anatomy of the Newborn*. New Haven: Yale University Press, 1973.

Jora, J. *Foot Reflexology: A Visual Guide for Self-Treatment*. New York: St. Martin's Press, 1991.

Kunz, B., and K. Kunz. *The Complete Guide to Foot Reflexology*. Albuquerque, NM: RRP Press, 2007.

Chapter 14: Crying, Fussing, and Other Baby Language

References

Acredolo, L., and S. Goodwyn. *Baby Signs: How to Talk with Your Baby Before Your Baby Can Talk*. Chicago: Contemporary Books, 1996.

Ainsworth, M., and S. Bell. "Infant crying and maternal responsiveness." *Child Development* 43 (1972).

Anisfeld, E., V. Casper, M. Nozyce, and N. Cunningham. "Does infant carrying promote attachment? An experimental study of the effects of increased physical contact on the development of attachment." *Child Development* 61 (1990).

Brazelton, T. *Learning to Listen: A Life Caring for Children*. Reading, MA: Perseus, 2013.

Brazelton, T., and J. Sparrow. *Calming Your Fussy Baby the Brazelton Way*. Reading, MA: Perseus, 2003.

Chisholm, J. S. "Swaddling, cradleboards, and the development of children." *Early Human Development* 2:3 (September 1978).

Clary, E., et al. "Socialization and situational influences on sustained altruism." *Child Development* 57 (1986).

Crockenberg, S. "Infant irritability, mother responsiveness, and social support influences in the security of infant-mother attachment." *Child Development* 52 (1981).

Cunningham, N., E. Anisfeld, V. Casper, and M. Nozyce. "Infant carrying, breast-feeding, and mother-infant relations: Cache or carry? Experimental evidence for positive effects of early infant carrying." *Lancet* 14 ((February 1987).

Gatts, J. D., et al. "Reduced crying and irritability in neonates using a continuously controlled early environment." *Infant Advantage: Clinical Reports,* 1995.

Gray, L., L. Watt, and E. M. Blass. "Skin-to-skin contact is analgesic in healthy newborns." *Pediatrics* 105:1 (January 2000): e14.

Guiney, J. B. *Read to Me, and I'll Teach You About . . . My Baby States.* Vienna, VA: Center for Infant & Family Resources, 2013.

Hunziker, U., and R. Barr. "Increased carrying reduces infant crying: A randomized controlled trial." *Pediatrics* 77:5 (May 1986).

Johanson, R. B., S. A. Spencer, P. Rolfe, P. Jones, and D. S. Massa. "Effect of post-delivery care on neonatal body temperature." *Acta Pediatrica* 81:11 (November 1992).

Karp, H. *The Happiest Baby on the Block: The New Way to Calm Crying and Help Your Newborn Baby Sleep Longer.* New York: Bantam Books, 2015.

Kopp, C. "A comparison of stimuli effective in soothing distressed infants." *Dissertation Abstracts* 31:12B (June 1971).

Korner, A., and E. Thoman. "The relative efficacy of contact and vestibular proprioceptive stimulation on soothing neonates." *Child Development* 43 (1972).

Levy, T. M., and M. Orlans. *Attachment, Trauma, and Healing: Understanding and Treating Attachment Disorder in Children and Families.* Washington, DC: CWLA Press, 1998.

MacFarlane, Jo. "Mothers who experience stress or worry before pregnancy 'more likely to have babies who cry for longer.'" DailyMail.com (September 6, 2014).

Moss, J., and H. C. Solomons. "Swaddling, then, there, and now: Historical, anthropological, and current practices." *Maternal Child Nursing* 8:3 (Fall 1979).

Murray, A. "Infant crying as an elicitor of parental behavior." *Psychological Bulletin* 86 (1979).

Roberts, M. "No language but a cry." *Psychology Today,* June 1987.

Sagi, A., and M. Hoffman. "Empathic distress in the newborn." *Developmental Psychology,* 1976.

Sears, W., and M. Sears. *Parenting the Fussy Baby and High-Need Child: Everything You Need to Know from Birth to Age Five.* Boston: Little, Brown, 1996.

Shaw, C. "A comparison of the patterns of mother-baby interactions for the group of crying, irritable babies and a group of more amenable babies." *Child Care, Health, and Development* 3 (1977).

Sherman, M. "Differentiation of emotional responses in infants: The ability of observers to judge the emotional characteristics of crying infants." *Journal of Comparative Psychology* 5 (1927).

Simner, M. "Newborn's responses to the cry of another infant." *Developmental Psychology* 5 (1971).

Solter, A. *The Aware Baby: A New Approach to Parenting.* Goleta, CA: Shining Star Press, 1984.

Wipfler, P. *Listening to Children: Crying.* Palo Alto, CA: Parents Leadership Institute, 1990.

Recommended Books

Jones, S. *Crying Baby, Sleepless Nights.* Boston: Harvard Common Press, 1992.

Karp, H. *The Happiest Baby on the Block: The New Way to Calm Crying and Help Your Newborn Baby Sleep Longer.* New York: Bantam Books, 2015.

Sears, W., and M. Sears. *Parenting the Fussy Baby and the High-Need Child: Everything You Need to Know from Birth to Age Five.* Boston: Little, Brown, 1996.

Simmons, W., and T. Brazelton. *The Self-Calmed Baby.* New York: St. Martin's Press, 1991.

Solter, A. *The Aware Baby: A New Approach to Parenting.* Goleta, CA: Shining Star Press, 2001.

———. *Tears and Tantrums: What to Do When Babies and Children Cry.* Goleta, CA: Shining Star Press, 1998.

Chapter 15: Minor Illness and Colic

References

Anderson, G. "Infant colic: A possible solution." *Maternal Child Nursing* 8 (1983).

Barr, R. G., S. J. McMullan, H. Spiess, et al. "Carrying as colic therapy: A randomized trial." *Pediatrics* 87 (1991).

Carey, W. "Maternal anxiety and infantile colic: Is there a relationship?" *Clinical Pediatrics* 31 (1968).

Craven, D. "Why colic?" *Medical Journal of Australia* 2 (1979).

Evans, R., et al. "Maternal diet and infantile colic in breastfed infants." *Lancet* 1 (1981).

Hsu, C. Y., et al. "Local massage after vaccination enhances the immunogenicity of diphtheria-tetanus-pertussis vaccine." *Pediatric Infectious Disease Journal* 14:7 (July 1995).

Jakobsson, L., and T. Lindberg. "Cow's milk proteins cause infantile colic in breastfed infants: A double blind study." *Pediatrics* 71 (1983).

Johanson, R. B., S. A. Spencer, P. Rofle, P. Jones, and D. S. Massa. "Effect of postdelivery care on neonatal body temperature." *Acta Pediatrica* 81:11 (November 1992).

Larsen, J. H. "Infants' colic and belly massage." *Practitioner* 234 (April 1990).

Liebman, W. "Infantile colic: Association with lactose and milk intolerance." *Journal of the American Medical Association* 245 (1981).

Lothe, L., et al. "Cow's milk formula as a cause of infantile colic: A double-blind study." *Pediatrics* 70 (1982).

Paradise, J. "Maternal and other factors in the etiology of infantile colic." *Journal of the American Medical Association* 197 (1966).

Said, G., et al. "Clinical trial of the treatment of colic by modification of parent-infant interaction." *Pediatrics* 74 (1984).

Sears, W., and M. Sears. *Parenting the Fussy Baby and the High-Need Child: Everything You Need to Know from Birth to Age Five.* Boston: Little, Brown, 1996.

Wessel, M., et al. "Paroxysmal fussing in infancy, sometimes called colic." *Pediatrics* 14 (1954).

Chapter 16: Your Premature Baby

References

Abdallah, B., L. K. Badr, and M. Hawaii. "The efficacy of massage on short- and long-term outcomes in preterm infants." *Infant and Child Development* 36:4 (2013): 662–69.

Affleck, G., J. H. Tennen, and J. Rowe. "Mothers, fathers, and the crisis of newborn intensive care." *Infant Mental Health Journal* 11:1 (1990).

Anisfeld, E., V. Casper, M. Nozyce, and N. Cunningham. "Does infant carrying promote attachment? An experimental study of the effects of increased physical contact on the development of attachment." *Child Development* 61 (1990).

Arnon, S., C. Diamant, S. Bauer, R. Regev, G. Sirota, and I. Litmanovitz. "Maternal singing during kangaroo care led to autonomic stability in preterm infants and reduced maternal anxiety." *Acta Pediatrica* 103:10 (2014): 1039–44.

Artese, C., and I. Blanchi. "Baby's messages to parents: Guide to the development of babies admitted to the NICU." European Foundation for the Care of Newborn Infants, 2014. www.efcni.org/fileadmin/Daten/Web/Newsletter/2014/2014 _April/Parents_guide_book_baby_s_messages_to_parents.pdf.

Bond, C. *The 5-Step Dialogue.* www.cherrybond.com.

Dunn, C., J. Sleep, and D. Collett. "Sensing an improvement: An experimental study to evaluate the use of aromatherapy, massage and periods of rest in an intensive care unit." *Journal of Advanced Nursing* 21:1 (January 1995).

Field, T. "Interventions for premature infants." *Journal of Pediatrics* 109 (1986).

Field, T., S. Schanberg, N. Gunzenhauser, and T. Brazelton. "Massage stimulates growth in preterm infants: A relocation." *Infant Behavior and Development* 13 (1990).

Field, T., S. Schanberg, F. Scafidi, C. Bauer, N. Vega-Lahr, R. Garcia, J. Nostrum, and C. Kuhn. "Cardiac and behavioral responses to repeated tactile and auditory stimulation of preterm and term neonates." *Developmental Psychology* 15 (July 1979).

———. "Tactile/kinesthetic stimulation effects on preterm neonates." *Pediatrics* 77 (May 1986).

Gottfried, A., et al. "Touch as an organizer for learning and development." In *The Many Facets of Touch,* ed. C. Brown et al. Johnson & Johnson Pediatric Round Table, no. 10. New York: Elsevier, 1980.

Grossman, K., et al. "Maternal tactual contact of the newborn after various postpartum conditions of mother-infant contact." *Developmental Psychology* 17 (March 1981).

Harrison, L. L., J. Leeper, and M. Yoon. "Effect of gentle human touch on preterm infants: Results from a pilot study." *Infant Behavior and Development* 15 (1990).

———. "Early parental touch and preterm infants." *Journal of Obstetric, Gynecologic, and Neonatal Nursing* 20:4 (1991).

———. "Effects of hospital-based instruction on interactions between parents and preterm infants." *Neonatal Network* 9:7 (1991).

———. "Preterm infants' physiologic responses early parent touch." *Western Journal of Nursing Research* 13:6 (1991).

Harrison, L. L., et al. "Effects of gentle human touch on preterm infants: Results from a pilot study." *Infant Behavior and Development* 15 (1992).

Heffernan, A., et al. "Baby massage—a teaching model." *Australian Nurses Journal* 13:6 (December-January 1984).

Heller, S. A. "A comparison of the effects of containment and stroking of preterm infants at varying levels of maturity." Ph.D. dissertation, Loyola University of Chicago, 1991.

Isaza, N. "Skin-to-skin contact with baby in neonatal unit decreases maternal stress levels: Already linked to happier, healthier newborns, study finds that snuggling with babies in intensive care eases mothers' anxiety that can interfere with parent-child bonding." *ScienceDaily,* October 23, 2015.

Johanson, R. B., S. A. Spencer, P. Rolfe, P. Jones, and D. S. Massa. "Effect of post-delivery care on neonatal body temperature." *Acta Pediatrica* 81:11 (November 1992).

Klaus, M., and A. Fanaroff. *Care of the High-risk Neonate.* Philadelphia: Saunders, 1986.

Kramer, M., et al. "Extra tactile stimulation of the premature infant." *Nursing Research* 24 (September-October 1975).

Kuhn, C. M., et al. "Tactile-kinesthetic stimulation effects on sympathetic and adrenocortical function in preterm infants." *Journal of Pediatrics* 119:3 (1981).

Macintosh, N. "Massage in preterm infants." *Archives of Disease in Childhood Fetal and Neonatal Education* 70:1 (January 1974).

McGrade, B. J., G. Affleck, D. Alen, and M. McQueeney. "Mothers of high-risk infants: Is their initial use of early intervention a predictor of later coping?" *Infant Mental Health Journal* 6:1 (1985).

Moses, H., and R. Phillips. "Skin hunger effects on preterm neonates." *Infant-Toddler Intervention* 6:1 (1996).

Oehler, J. "The development of the preterm infant's responsiveness to auditory and tactile social stimuli." *Dissertation Abstracts* 45:8B (February 1985).

Paterson, L. "Baby massage in the neonatal unit." *Nursing: Journal of Clinical Practice, Education and Management* 4:23 (November-December 1990).

Powell, L. "The effect of extra stimulation and maternal involvement on the development of low birthweight infants and on maternal behavior." *Child Development* 45 (March 1974).

Rausch, P. "Effects of tactile and kinesthetic stimulation on premature infants." *Journal of Obstetric, Gynecological, and Neonatal Nursing* 10:1 (1981).

———. "A tactile and kinesthetic stimulation program for premature infants." In *The Many Facets of Touch*, ed. C. Brown et al. Johnson & Johnson Pediatric Round Table, no. 10. New York: Elsevier, 1984.

Rice, R. "Premature infants respond to sensory stimulation." *APA Monitor,* November 1975.

———. "Cardiac and behavioral responsivity to tactile stimulation in premature and full term infants." *Developmental Psychology* 12:4 (July 1976).

———. "Neurophysiological development in premature infants." *Developmental Psychology* 12:4 (July 1976).

Rose, S. "Effects of prematurity and early intervention on responsiveness to tactual stimuli: A comparison of term and preterm infants." *Child Development* 51:2 (June 1980).

———. "Preterm responses to passive, active, and social touch." In *The Many Facets of Touch*, ed. C. Brown et al. Johnson & Johnson Pediatric Round Table, no. 10. New York: Elsevier, 1984.

Scafidi, F., et al. "Effects of tactile/kinesthetic stimulation on the clinical course and sleep/wake behavior of preterm neonates." *Infant Behavior and Development* 9:1 (January 1986).

———. "Massage stimulates growth in preterm infants: A replication." *Infant Behavior and Development* 13 (1990).

Schaeffer, J. "The effects of gentle human touch on mechanically ventilated very short gestation infants." *Maternal Child Nursing* [Monograph 12], vol. 11 (1982).

Stern, M., et al. "Prematurity stereotyping: Effects on mother-infant interaction." *Child Development* 57:2 (April 1986).

Walt, J., et al. "Mother-infant interactions at two and three months in preterm SGA, and full term infants." *Early Human Development*, September 1985.

Wang, L., J. L. He, and X. H. Zhang. "The efficacy of massage on preterm infants: A meta-analysis." *American Journal of Perinatology* 30:9 (October 2013): 731–38.

Warren, I., and C. Bond. *A Guide to Infant Development in the Newborn Nursery,* 5th ed. London: Early Babies, 2010.

———. *Caring for Your Baby in the Neonatal Unit: A Parent's Handbook*. London: Early Babies, 2015.

White, J., et al. "The effects of tactile and kinesthetic stimulation on neonatal development in the premature infants." *Developmental Psychobiology* 9 (November 1976).

World Health Organization. "Preterm birth." Fact sheet no. 363, November 2015. www.who.int\mediacentre\factsheets\fs363.

White-Trait, R. C., and M. N. Goldman. "Maternally administered tactile, auditory, visual and vestibular stimulation: Relationship to later interactions between mothers and premature infants." *Research in Nursing and Health* 11 (1988).

Recommended Books

Downing, C. R. *Premature Grandpa: A Science Guy's Experience in the NICU with His Granddaughter*. CRD Press, 2015.

Garcia-Prats, J., and S. Hornfischer. *What to Do When Your Baby Is Premature: A Parent's Handbook for Coping with High Risk Pregnancy and Caring for the Preterm Infant*. New York: Three Rivers Press, 2000.

Gunter, J. *The Preemie Primer: A Complete Guide for Parents of Premature Babies—from Birth Through the Toddler Years and Beyond*. Philadelphia: Da Capo Press, 2010.

Linden, D. W., E. T. Paroli, and M. W. Doron. *Preemies: The Essential Guide for Parents of Premature Babies,* 2nd ed. New York: Gallery Books, 2010.

Madden, S. *The Preemie Parents' Companion: The Essential Guide to Caring for Your Premature Baby in the Hospital, at Home, and Through the First Years*. Boston: Harvard Common Press, 2000.

Sears, W., R. Sears, J. Sears, and M. Sears. *The Premature Baby Book: Everything You Need to Know About Your Premature Baby from Birth to Age One*. Boston: Little, Brown, 2004.

Chapter 17: Your Baby with Special Needs

References

Als, H., et al. "Stages of early behavioral organization: The study of a sighted infant and a blind infant in interaction with their mothers." In *High Risk Infants and Children: Adult and Peer Interactions*. New York: Academic Press, 1980.

Ayres, J. *Sensory Integration and the Child: Understanding Hidden Sensory Challenges*. Los Angeles: Western Psychological Services, 2005.

Bigelow, A. "The development of reaching in blind infants." *British Journal of Developmental Psychology* 4 (November 1988).

Bushnell, E. "Relationship between visual and tactual exploration by six-motholds." *Developmental Psychology* 21:4 (July 1985).

Clark, L. "The importance of touch with an anencephalic baby." *Maternal Child Nursing* 7:5 (September-October 1982).

Cratty, B., and T. Sams. *The Body Image of Blind Children*. New York: American Foundation for the Blind, 1968.

Drehobl, K., and M. Fuhr. *Pediatric Massage for the Child with Special Needs*. Tucson, AZ: Therapy Skill Builders, 2000.

Fraser, B. "Child Impairment and Parent-Infant Communication." *Child Care, Health, and Development* 12 (1986).

Geralis, E. *Children with Cerebral Palsy: A Parent's Guide*. Bethesda, MD: Woodbine House, 1998.

Gregory, S. "Mother speech to young hearing impaired children." *Journal of the British Association of Teachers of the Deaf* 3 (1979).

Hansen, R. "Motorically impaired infants: Impact of a massage procedure on caregiver-infant interactions." *Journal of the Multihandicapped Person* 1:1 (1988).

Hart, V. "Characteristics of young blind children." Paper presented at the Second International Symposium on Visually Handicapped Infants and Young Children: Birth to Seven, Aruba, 1983.

Heller, M., and E. Gentaz. *Psychology of Touch and Blindness*. New York: Psychology Press, 2014.

Infant Hearing Resource. *Parent-Infant Communication: A Program of Clinical and Home Training for Parents and Hearing Impaired Infants*. Portland, OR: Infant Hearing Resource, 1985.

Korner, A., et al. "Visual alertness in neonates as evoked by maternal care." *Journal of Experimental Child Psychology* 10 (1970).

Linkous, L. W. and R. M. Stutts. "Passive tactile stimulation effects on the muscle tone of hypotonic, developmentally delayed young children." *Perceptual and Motor Skills,* 71:3, 1990.

Meyer, D., ed. *Uncommon Fathers: Reflections on Raising a Child with a Disability*. Bethesda, MD: Woodbine House, 1995.

Niemann, S., and N. Jacob. *Helping Children Who are Blind: Family and Community Support for Children with Vision Problems*. Berkeley, CA: Hesperian Foundation, 2000.

Porter, S. J. "The use of massage for neonates requiring special care." *Complementary Therapies in Nursing and Midwifery,* August 1996.

Riesen, A. "Sensory Deprivation." In *Progress in Physiological Psychology,* ed. E. Stellar and J. Sprague. New York: Academic Press, 1966.

Rutter, N. "Response of term babies to a warm environment." *Archives of the Disabled Child* 53 (March 1979).

Scaridi, F., and T. Field. "Massage therapy improves behavior in neonates born to HIV-positive mothers." *Journal of Pediatric Psychology* 21:6 (December 1996).

Sears, W., R. Sears, J. Sears, and M. Sears. *The Premature Baby Book: Everything*

You Need to Know About Your Premature Baby from Birth to Age One. Boston: Little, Brown, 2004.

Simons, R. *After the Tears: Parents Talk About Raising a Child with a Disability.* New York: Harcourt Brace, 1998.

Slater, C. "Massaging crack babies." *Massage Magazine* 28 (1990).

Speirer, J. *Infant Massage for Developmentally Delayed Babies.* Denver, CO: United Cerebral Palsy Center, 1982.

———. *Therapeutic Infant Massage as an Intervention for Parent and Child Attachment.* Denver, CO: United Cerebral Palsy Center, 1982.

Strauss, L. "The effects of tactile stimulation on the communicative, social-emotional, and motor behaviors of deaf-blind-multi-handicapped infants." *Dissertation Abstracts* 42:10A (April 1982).

Warren, D. *Blindness and Early Childhood Development.* New York: American Foundation for the Blind, 1984.

Weber, K. "Massage for drug exposed infants." *Massage Therapy Journal,* Summer 1991.

Wheaten, A., F. A. Scaridi, T. Field, G. Ironson, C. Valdeon, and E. Bandstra. "Massage effects on cocaine-exposed preterm neonates." *Journal of Developmental and Behavioral Pediatrics* 14:5 (1993).

White, B., and R. Held. "Plasticity of sensorimotor development in the human infant." In *Causes of Behavior: Readings in Child Development and Educational Psychology,* 2d ed., ed. J. Rosenblith and W. Allinsmith. Boston: Allyn & Bacon, 1966.

Wills, D. "The ordinary devoted mother and her blind baby." *Psychoanalytic Study of the Child* 34 (1979).

Zimmerman, J. "Social interaction patterns between blind and multi-impaired infants and their mothers: An analysis." *Dissertation Abstracts* 42:7A (1982).

Recommended Books

Behrman, R. E. *The Future of Children: Drug Exposed Infants.* New York: Center for the Future of Children, 1991.

Bull, M. T. *Keys to Parenting a Child with Down Syndrome.* New York: Barron's, 1993.

Geralis, E., ed. *Children with Cerebral Palsy: A Parent's Guide.* Bethesda, MD: Woodbine House, 1998.

Hale, N. *Down Syndrome Parenting 101: Must-Have Advice for Making Your Life Easier.* Bethesda, MD: Woodbine House, 2011.

Heller, M., and E. Gentaz. *Psychology of Touch and Blindness.* New York: Psychology Press, 2014.

Hollbrook, M., ed. *Children with Visual Impairments: A Parent's Guide.* Bethesda, MD: Woodbine House, 1996.

Hughes, S. *What Makes Ryan Tick? A Family's Triumph over Tourette Syndrome and Attention Deficiency Hyperactivity Disorder.* Duarte, CA: Hope Press, 1996.

Kephart, B. A. *A Slant of Sun: One Child's Courage.* New York: W. W. Norton, 1998.

Kranowitz, C., and L. Silver. *The Out-of-Sync Child: Recognizing and Coping with Sensory Processing Disorder.* New York: Penguin Group, 2005.

Kumin, L. *Early Communication Skills for Children with Down Syndrome: A Guide for Parents and Professionals.* Bethesda, MD: Woodbine House, 2003.

Meyer, D. J., ed. *Uncommon Fathers: Reflections on Raising a Child with a Disability.* Bethesda, MD: Woodbine House, 1995.

Sacks, O. *Seeing Voices: A Journey into the World of the Deaf.* New York: Harper, 2000.

Shapiro, L. *Uncommon Voyage: Parenting a Special Needs Child in the World of Alternative Medicine.* London: Faber and Faber, 2001.

Simons, J. *The Down Syndrome Transition Handbook: Charting Your Child's Course to Adulthood.* Bethesda, MD: Woodbine House, 2010.

Simons, R. *After the Tears: Parents Talk About Raising a Child with a Disability.* New York: Harcourt Brace, 1998.

Skallerup, S. *Babies with Down Syndrome: A New Parents' Guide.* Bethesda, MD: Woodbine House, 2008.

Stray-Gundersen, K. *Babies with Down Syndrome: A New Parents' Guide.* Bethesda, MD: Woodbine House, 2012.

Sumar, S. *Yoga for the Special Child: A Therapeutic Approach for Infants and Children with Down Syndrome, Cerebral Palsy, and Learning Disabilities.* New York: Buckingham, 1998. Website: www.specialyoga.com

Warren, D. *Blindness and Early Childhood Development.* New York: American Foundation for the Blind, 1984.

Chapter 18: Your Growing Child
and Sibling Bonding Through Massage

References

Karen, R. *Becoming Attached: First Relationships and How They Shape Our Capacity to Love.* New York: Oxford University Press, 1998.

Montague, A. *Touching: The Human Significance of the Skin.* New York: Oxford University Press, 1998.

Zacher Laves, C. U. "Suggestions for adaptations of the massage with the growing child." Private communication to author, 1999.

Recommended Books

Cole, J., S. Calmenson, and A. Tiegreen. *Pat-a-Cake and Other Play Rhymes.* New York: Morrow, 1992.

Staff, T., and G. Mohrmann. *1001 Rhymes and Fingerplays.* Boston: Watten, 2001.

Chapter 19: Your Adopted or Foster Children

References

Acredolo, L., and S. Goodwyn. *Baby Signs: How to Talk to Your Baby Before Your Baby Can Talk*. Chicago: Contemporary Books, 2009.

Bacchetta, S. *What I Want My Adopted Child to Know*. iUniverse, 2010.

Bond, J. "Post adoption depression syndrome." *ADOPT*: Assistance Information Support, Spring 1995, www.adopting.org.

Clark, S. "Prenatal Trauma and the Adoptee Experience." *Pact, An Adoption Alliance*, 1995, www.pactadopt.org.

Dubucs, R. "Touching and the adopted child." *International Concerns for Children*, 1998.

Hage, D. "Foundations of Attachment." *International Concerns for Children*, 1999.

Henning, R. S. Personal letter to author, 1999.

Ingram, J. "Russian Foster Families Face Huge Task." *Philadelphia Inquirer*, December 18, 1998.

Karen, R. *Becoming Attached: First Relationships and How They Shape Our Capacity to Love*. New York: Oxford University Press, 1998.

Kurson, B. "Foster parents face a life of rough breaks." *Chicago Sun Times*, March 14, 1999.

Melina, L. "Attachment to older child has some twists." *Adopted Child*, January 1985.

———. "Unattached child: Going through life not caring." *Adopted Child*, February 1985.

———. "Attachment theorists believe parent-infant experiences determine later behavior." *Adopted Child*, May 1997.

Russell, M. "The lifelong impact of adoption." *Pact, An Adoption Alliance*, 1998, www.pactadopt.org.

Singer, L., et al. "Mother-infant attachment: How does adoption affect a newborn?" *Pact, An Adoption Alliance*, 1998, www.pactadopt.org.

Steinberg, G. "Bonding and attachment: How does adoption affect a newborn?" *Pact, An Adoption Alliance*, 1998, www.pactadopt.org.

"The special love of foster parents." *Record Online*, December 6, 1998.

Verrier, N. *The Primal Wound: Understanding the Adopted Child*. Baltimore: Gateway Press, 2003.

Recommended Books

Babb, L., R. Laws, and R. DeBolt. *Adopting and Advocating for the Special Needs Child*. Westport, CT: Bergin & Garvey, 1997.

Canfield, J., M. Hansen, H. McNamara, and K. Simmons. *Chicken Soup for the Soul: Children with Special Needs*. Deerfield Beach, FL: Health Communications, 2012.

Davis, S. *Do You Want to Be a Foster Parent?* Sausalito, CA: Lucid Press, 1998.

Johnson, N. *Adoption Book for Parents: Everything You Should Know About Adopting Your First Child*. N. Johnson, 2014.

Karen, R. *Becoming Attached: First Relationships and How They Shape Our Capacity to Love*. New York: Oxford University Press, 1999.

Keck, G., and R. Kupecky. *Adopting the Hurt Child: Hope for Families with Special-Needs Kids*. Colorado Springs, CO: NavPress, 2009.

Kasky, R., and J. Kasky. *99 Things You Wish You Knew Before Choosing Adoption*. Florida, NY: 99 Series, 2012.

Melina, L. *Raising Adopted Children*. New York: HarperPerennial, 1998.

Russell, M. *Adoption Wisdom: A Guide to the Issues and Feelings of Adoption*. Santa Monica, CA: Broken Branch Productions, 2010.

Verrier, N. *The Primal Wound: Understanding the Adopted Child*. Baltimore: Gateway Press, 2003.

Chapter 20: A Note to Teen Parents

References

Crockenberg, S. B. "Professional support for adolescent mothers: Who gives it, how adolescent mothers evaluate it, what they would prefer." *Infant Mental Health Journal* 4:1 (1986).

Field, T., S. Widmayer, S. Adler, and M. de Cubas. *Teenage Parenting in Different Cultures, Family Constellations, and Caregiving Environments: Effects on Infant Development*. Miami: University of Miami Medical School, 1986.

Herzog, E. P., D. S. Cherniss, and B. J. Menzel. "Issues in engaging high-risk adolescent mothers in supportive work." *Infant Mental Health Journal* 7:1 (1986).

Jamiolkowski, R. *A Baby Doesn't Make the Man: Alternative Sources of Power and Manhood for Young Men*. New York: Rosen Publishing Group, 1997.

Siegel, D. *Brainstorm: The Power and Purpose of the Teenage Brain*. New York: Penguin, 2013.

Recommended Books

Biegel, G. *The Stress Reduction Workbook for Teens: Mindfulness Skills to Help You Deal with Stress*. Oakland, CA: New Harbinger Publications, 2009.

Gore, A. *The Hip Mama Survival Guide*. New York: Hyperion, 1998.

———. *The Mother Trip: Hip Mama's Guide to Staying Sane in the Chaos of Motherhood*. Seattle, WA: Seal Press 2000.

Goyer, T. *Teen Mom: You're Stronger than You Think*. Grand Rapids, MI: Zondervan, 2015.

Hart, S. *The Essential Teen Pregnancy Guide*. Benjamin Sweet, 2015.

Jamiolkowski, R. *A Baby Doesn't Make the Man: Alternative Sources of Power and Manhood for Young Men*. New York: Rosen Publishing Group, 2001.

Lerman, E., and J. Moffett. *Teen Moms: The Pain and the Promise*. Buena Park, CA: Morning Glory Press 1997.

Lindsay, J., and J. Brunelli. *Your Pregnancy and Newborn Journey: A Guide for Pregnant Teens.* Buena Park, CA: Morning Glory Press, 2004.

Morris, J. *Road to Fatherhood: How to Help Young Dads Become Loving and Responsible Parents.* Buena Park, CA: Morning Glory Press, 2002.

Siegel, D. *Brainstorm: The Power and Purpose of the Teenage Brain.* New York: Penguin, 2013.

Simpson, C. *Coping with Teenage Motherhood.* New York: Rosen Publishing Group, 1997.

Trapani, M. *Listen Up: Teenage Mothers Speak Out.* New York: Rosen Publishing Group, 1997.

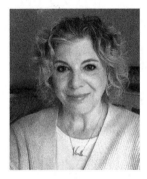

Vimala McClure is the founder of the International Association of Infant Massage, a nonprofit organization with instructors in more than seventy countries. Her groundbreaking first book, *Infant Massage: A Handbook for Loving Parents,* brought the ancient practice of infant massage to the West and has been translated into many languages. She has had the great fortune of working in Mother Teresa's Nirmala Shishu Bhavan (baby hospital) in Kolkata, India. During the 1990s she pursued fiber arts and became an award-winning quilt artist. She has been practicing yoga and meditation since 1970. She lives in Boulder Colorado, her "ancestral home."

vimalaji@comcast.net
About.me/vimalamcclure
vimalaji.wordpress.com
IAIM International newsletter: iaim.net